Diary of a Medical Intuitive

One Woman's Eye-Opening Journey
from No-Nonsense E.R. Nurse to
Open-Hearted Healer and Visionary

Christel Nani, RN, Ph.D.

L.M. PRESS
Cayucos, California

L. M. PRESS
P.O. Box 345, Cayucos, CA 93430
(805) 545-0888
fax (805) 435-1472
www.LMPress.com – info@LMPress.com

Editor: Margot Silk Forrest
www.margotsilkforrest.com
Cover Design: Peri Poloni, Knockout Designs
www.knockoutbooks.com

Publisher's Cataloguing-in-Publication Data
Nani, Christel
    Diary of a Medical Intuitive: One Woman's Eye-Opening Jour-
ney from No-Nonsense E.R. Nurse to Open-Hearted Healer and
Visionary / Christel Nani. – 1ˢᵗ ed.
    p. cm.
    Includes index.
ISBN: 0-9741450-2-5

Also by Christel Nani:

Guidance 24/7
How to Open Your Heart and Let Angels Into Your Life

Two Frequently Asked Questions

Why Would I Use a Medical Intuitive?

A reputable Medical Intuitive can quickly identify the true cause of your symptoms, both at the physical level and at the emotional/spiritual level where illness has its roots. This is why most people consult a Medical Intuitive, and it's probably why you picked up this book.

In addition, an energy scan by a Medical Intuitive can identify any vulnerable points in your body (or spirit) where disease could take hold in the future. This is because all illness shows up as a block in your energy system *before* it invades your body. Medical Intuitives are like an elegant early-warning system, the best kind of preventive medicine.

Finally — and this is something most people don't know — a Medical Intuitive can tell you what's blocking your "health" in terms of relationships, career, and finances. The causes of "illness" in these areas are also apparent in your energy system. Many business people, actors, and entertainers have come to me for a reading to determine what's in the way of finding the right partner, bumping up their career a notch, or having their business take off.

Do I Have to Believe in It for It to Work?

Absolutely not. I do use a number of special terms and concepts in this book (such as energy field, energetic signature, vibration, resonance, and magnetics) to explain how and why medical intuition works. But *anyone* can be successfully diagnosed by a reputable Medical Intuitive, whether you believe in these concepts or not. If your own belief system is different than mine, medical intuition can still be a tremendous force for good in your life. The same is true if you want to go one step further and not just discover the cause of your suffering but put an end to it.

Christel Nani

To my grandmother Tessie

Thank you for teaching me that there is a hero

within each of us and that humor

can be found anywhere.

Table of Contents

viii

Foreword

By Rebecca Grace, Psy.D.

Usually the foreword of a book is written by a famous person who doesn't really know the author, but who has agreed to lend their name to give the book credence or popularity.

Well, I am not famous. I am a psychologist who was leading a very active and productive life until being struck down by multiple sclerosis in 1999. Within months, I was looking at life in a wheelchair – or worse. When I finally gave up on Western medicine, I turned to Christel Nani, and I was healed because of her work. I am not in remission. My MS is not "under control." I am healed. Fully healed, despite the fact that medical authorities say MS is incurable. This is what qualifies me to write the foreword to this book.

I first met Christel over the phone, some time before I became ill. I was making arrangements with her to do a reading for my mother, who had just been diagnosed with Stage IV terminal cancer. A client of mine, upon hearing of my mom's illness, had given me Christel's name, and my mother eagerly agreed to a

1

reading. She was not seeking healing, though. She simply wanted peace of mind at the end of her life.

To this day I do not know everything that Christel and my mother talked about. I only know that from their first conversation, my mother began to change – and change dramatically. A light that had gone out in her decades before returned, and burned brighter and brighter up to the moment of her passing two months later.

I was amazed at what this mysterious woman had done for my mother. My mom loved talking with Christel, never argued with her (much to my amazement), and followed all her instructions to the letter. My mother was done with this life, so physical longevity was not something she desired or sought, but she left this planet with a peace, serenity, and purpose that inspire me to this day. I must admit to having been being a bit offended, that I, a highly successful psychologist, could not help my mom in the way that this stranger had – and all on the phone. They never met in person.

After my mom's death, I called Christel to thank her for everything she had done for my mom and my whole family. Mom had a good passing, and it particularly helped my elderly father, whose heart was broken at losing her. At the end of our conversation, Christel mentioned that if I ever wanted a reading myself, she would be happy to do one. I thought, "That's great, but she works with sick people and I'm never sick."

Over the next few months, I referred a number of my psychotherapy clients who were dealing with physical ailments to Christel. Every one of them came back with what I considered to be a profound insight or new awareness. We would then work in therapy on what they'd discovered, and wonderful changes resulted. I was deeply impressed, but also a little threatened at how this woman could know so much about people – and help them understand themselves so quickly — with no prior knowledge of them. It was mysterious and puzzling to me. It also shook my foundations as a psychologist: I saw that psychological testing and long interviews with new clients yielded little truly useful information compared with a single reading by Christel. I also saw that Christel's ability to name the one priority task a person needs to focus on was a profound gift. When completed, this task — invariably one of emotional or spiritual growth — would untangle a myriad of other problems quietly and easily. At this point, I still had not met Christel face to face, but her work continued to amaze me.

A few months after my mom's death, I began to experience an array of frightening and puzzling symptoms. Chalking it up to stress, I took a weekend away in the mountains, a place that has always restored my spirit. However, instead of hiking with great energy as I used to, I had difficulty even walking. This continued when I returned home. For some reason, my legs were no longer obeying my commands to move smoothly and easily. A weird numbness and other sensations started appearing not only in my legs but in other parts of my body as well. I began running into door jambs. My balance suddenly seemed off. It was clear I had to seek medical care.

As many people with illness have found out, Western medicine is sometimes sadly lacking in adequate or thoughtful care. Shortly after my entry into the world of doctors, sophisticated and sometimes painful tests, and long waits, I knew that this path would only hasten my slide into sickness. I prayed for guidance, and Christel's name came instantly to mind.

My first appointment with Christel was memorable, to say the least. I was angry, confused, frustrated, and frightened about what was happening to me. I didn't tell her about my symptoms or concerns, though. I just sat down and she started her reading.

I don't remember all that she told me, I only know I felt a shiver of recognition at the truth of her words. I know now that this shiver was my soul celebrating the knowledge that it had finally been heard.

Here are some of the snippets I do remember. Christel asked, "Have you had your brain scanned?"(In some cases, plaque in the brain is evident and confirms the presence of .) She told me, "Not all parts of your brain are talking to all parts of your body," and said, "I find that in your etheric field you have the resonance of multiple sclerosis."

I didn't know exactly what some of these terms meant, but I was shocked by what I heard. This woman knew nothing about me, yet she knew everything. (My physician had suspected MS from the start, though at this point I had not completed a full diagnostic workup.) This woman also knew things I didn't want to know, couldn't accept, and tried frantically to argue with. She knew how afraid I was, how very sick I would become, and what I needed to change in order to get well.

My soul told me I needed to work with Christel, but I really wasn't a very nice patient. I think she dreaded me coming as much as I dreaded going. For a few months I really fought her. I am profoundly grateful she followed her guidance not to "fire" me, and I'm grateful I followed mine to keep trying. However, my stubbornness resulted in me becoming quite ill. Some people have to practically become road kill to get motivated to do their inner work. Unfortunately, I was one of them.

Over time, though, I softened and became willing to accept what she said to me and to do her suggested assignments. There were many difficult times because I had to confront the shadow in me that remained despite my professional training and the psychotherapy I had done. But there is a profound difference between awareness and healing, and I was learning it. I think being a psychologist actually hampered my healing work at first. Thank God I was able to get over myself!

About a year and half after becoming ill, I had a spontaneous healing while lying on the table where Christel did hands-on healing. I suddenly experienced a moment in time when nothing was left in me to fight or to be stubborn. After that instant, I had a miraculous turnaround. My physical energy returned immediately. Twenty-four hours later, I used my cane for the last time. Over the next eleven months, every single symptom I'd had unwound itself, leaving in the exact order in which they came.

I have been well ever since – well in body and spirit and deeply, deeply happy. Since my healing, I have had the privilege of working closely with Christel to found the Center for Spiritual Responsibility, teach the principles of healing, and help people make choices that align with their souls. I am still amazed at Christel's gift for reading people and knowing exactly what will heal their illness, whether their suffering is physical, emotional or spiritual.

A few last words before you embark on the journey of discovery embodied in this book. Christel is the most penetratingly honest person I have ever known. It is impossible to lie to her; she compels you to know your truth. Her spiritual connection and ongoing communication with God inspire me. She has an unwavering willingness to be responsible for her own feelings and actions, and she absolutely walks her talk. She is a spiritual teacher, a powerful woman, and a gifted healer. I cannot count how many people have called me to thank me for referring them to Christel and have added, "She's the real thing, you know."

I have seen people heal things that modern medicine says can't be healed, whether it's a serious illness or a personality disorder. I have seen firsthand the miracles that happen when someone is willing to consider what Christel tells them and take the suggested actions.

We all know that there is a mind-body connection, that our thoughts affect our lives in profound ways. What Christel does is to give people a road map showing exactly which thoughts are hurting them, what is causing these thoughts, and how to change them. Her heart's desire is to promote a grassroots movement, a revolution where people will be able to make choices that make them happy, free of unconscious baggage and loyalty to old ideas. This book is the story of her personal journey to freedom and healing, and her vision for a future where individuals raise the spiritual level of the entire planet simply by being profoundly happy.

I am honored to work with her, to be her friend, and to join with her in showing people what can happen when they listen to their souls. I am excited that you will get to experience the miracle of Christel's gift. Jesus said, "What I can do, you can do also." He wasn't kidding.

I wish you health, inspiration, and the courage to make living in alignment with your soul more important than your fears.

Rebecca Grace
Encinitas, California
February 20, 2004
The third anniversary of my spontaneous healing

CHAPTER 1

Birth of a New York Skeptic

Skepticism rants and raves or raises a chilly eyebrow
while Reality patiently stands there, waiting
for all the fuss to die down.

When I was eight years old, I suddenly realized two things: Our neighbor was about to die, and I would be an emergency-room nurse when I grew up. I had no reason to doubt or fear this sudden knowledge, but I did learn a valuable cautionary lesson from it. There are certain things that one should not bring up at the dinner table.

Our neighbor, an apparently healthy man in his fifties, was a local policeman and a great buddy of mine. He always called me Charlie instead of Christel because I was a passionate tomboy. My loving nickname for him was Mr. Oatmeal.

One warm summer evening he and his wife were standing in our backyard laughing with my parents. When I banged open the screen door and went outside to join them, I saw something was wrong. His skin seemed a funny color, and he didn't look quite as solid as he should have. I didn't analyze it – I was just eight, after all – but I knew quite clearly that my buddy was going to die very soon.

My foreknowledge didn't feel sad – I simply understood that Mr. Oatmeal was leaving and it was his time to go. To me it seemed completely natural. When I casually shared this information with my family over dinner that night, they were shocked and distressed – not that Mr. Oatmeal was going to die, of course, but that I should think such a thing. I couldn't explain that it was not something I thought, but something I *knew*.

When he suddenly died three days later, everyone was stunned by it. My parents were too shocked to say anything about my prediction of his death. It became the proverbial elephant in the living room that no one talks about. Weeks later, my mom took me aside and said I shouldn't think about negative things, only positive things, and that I should never *ever* talk about someone dying again. My prescience scared them silly.

As for me, I wasn't scared. I was *terrified*. We had always been taught that having bad thoughts about a person could make them come true. Had I made my friend Mr. Oatmeal die?

A deep fear of intuition was born in me that day. It was nurtured by a short but unforgettable stint in Catholic school, where we learned that clairvoyance was associated with evil and anyone who claimed to be psychic was a tool of the devil. And that was even before my devoutly Catholic mother grabbed my brother's new Ouija board, marched it out the back door, and flung it into the garbage can after she found us trying to contact our long-dead grandfather with it.

I was nine by then, and someone had given my older brother a Ouija board for his birthday. With it you could supposedly get messages from the spirits of people who had died. You simply placed your hands on a glass indicator that would move – apparently by itself – pausing over letters printed on the board to spell out the answers to the questions.

We had played with the board before, but our mother didn't pay much attention. That afternoon, we wanted to know what the future would bring, and we decided to ask our grandfather, who had died two years earlier. We posed our question and placed our four grubby little hands on the glass indicator. It started moving immediately. We laughed out loud – it seemed to take on a life of its own. Quickly it spelled out a response. "I am glad to talk to you," it told us.

We said, "Are you our grandfather?" But the answer was "NO!" It came so quickly, jerking our arms abruptly from the N to the O to the exclamation point, that we jumped back from the board involuntarily.

Just then our mother walked into the room. She assessed the situation in a nanosecond, grabbed the Ouija board and the mysterious glass indicator, and headed for the back door.

"You are never to touch that *thing* again!" she shouted. "Do you hear me? It's evil, and it's dangerous!"

Eyes wide, we nodded – and waited until nightfall to retrieve the board and hide it in the shed. It was dangerous and therefore exciting. We continued playing with the forbidden Ouija board in secret, but our mother's sudden fury had left us scared, bewildered, and very clear on the concept that trying to contact spirits was bad. Catholic children did not do such things.

Two years later, my family was celebrating Labor Day with a barbeque in a neighbor's yard. Some people were eating hamburgers and potato salad; the rest of us were playing a marathon game of badminton, which I loved. That afternoon, however, I let the birdie drop at my feet. An uncomfortable sensation had shot through my body. It felt as if I'd been kicked in the stomach by a horse. My teammates called my name. The world slowed until it seemed like I was very far away listening to the sounds of the barbeque but not really there. I felt like I was floating through the air, unattached to my body. I saw everyone and heard everything from a distance, but I was clearly elsewhere. I enjoyed the sensation until I saw a vision. My three-year-old brother, Stephen, was lying on his back, eyes open, in a serene but very lifelike pose. There wasn't a mark on him, but he was clearly dead. He seemed to be floating in the sky.

I'm told I screamed his name, and the world suddenly went into overdrive. Everyone was calling Stephen's name, searching the back and front yards. I was terrified. I didn't understand what the vision meant, but I sure knew what it looked like. People raced out to the street, fearing the worst but not finding my brother.

Suddenly I understood the vision. "He's floating," I screamed. In the chaos, only one person seemed to hear me: Stephen's godmother. She ran to our backyard and headed straight for our above-ground pool. Someone had left the ladder down. She climbed up and saw Stephen, eyes wide open, arms stretched toward the sky, floating serenely, but not breathing. She pulled him out and coaxed the breath back into him as my mother wept.

When Stephen's godmother was asked how she knew to look for him in the pool, she said she'd heard a voice inside of her head. She couldn't identify that voice as mine.

As for me, I was so shaken and terrified by my part in all this, I said nothing about it. I put the whole experience out of my mind. The years rolled by. I went to junior high, then high school. The popular culture of the day looked on psychic abilities as a joke, and I hopped on the bandwagon – until the day six years later when I got my driver's license.

To celebrate the big event I took Stephen to the store for a treat. He was nine and I was seventeen. I was waiting near the counter and Stephen was happily buying candy when I started getting that far-away feeling again. The world slowed, and I felt like I was floating above it all. From that viewpoint, I watched in horror as Stephen walked out of the store and directly into the path of a car that had seemingly come from nowhere. Stephen had frozen and the car was bearing down upon him when I shook myself back to the present. I yelled his name. Stephen had left the store and, preoccupied with his goodies, had absentmindedly stepped from the curb into the street.

I ran after him screaming, "Stop! Stop!" Stephen stopped in mid-stride and turned to look at me just as a car drove directly into his path. I heard the screech of the brakes and saw the paleness of the driver's face as he narrowly missed my little brother.

Shaken doesn't begin to describe the effect of the adrenalin rush from watching your youngest brother almost die. Then and there I chose to pay attention to my visions, waking or sleeping. I read up on people who had portents of danger and how helpful this foreknowledge could be. I also learned that the messenger was usually beheaded when the information wasn't good.

Then denial took over again. My logical mind interrupted my research. This can't be real, it said. So I dismissed the truth and explained away all the extrasensory experiences I'd had. I proceeded to act (consciously and unconsciously) as if they'd never happened.

Bear in mind that part of my innate skepticism came from the fact that I grew up in New York, a place that often makes fun of anything even faintly weird or woo-woo. I joined the crowd in dismissing with a sophisticated sneer the powers of psychics, mediums, intuitives, and clairvoyants. No one could see the future, and anyone who claimed she could was either fooling herself, faking it, or genuinely evil.

This stance didn't stop my intuitive abilities from developing, however. I kept having "experiences" (I didn't know what else to call them), though I never talked to anyone about them again. While I could easily dismiss such phenomena in others, I had to work harder and harder to ignore, discount, or deny them in myself.

Eventually I entered college, immersed myself in my studies, and became the committed emergency-room nurse I had known I would be all those years ago. I dedicated myself to the world of Western medicine, the world of science and empirical proof. If you wanted me to believe something, you had to prove it to me. If I couldn't see it, touch it, smell it, or taste it, it wasn't real. I was a full-fledged New York skeptic – and proud of it.

CHAPTER 2

Adventures in the E.R.

When something looks like a duck, walks like a duck, and
quacks like the duck, eventually we have to admit it is a duck.

Studying medicine is a good pursuit for skeptics. Hard science satisfied my need for facts, formulas, and forthright answers to complex problems. It also gave me a wealth of information I could use to logically explain (to myself) how I instantly knew what was wrong with the people who came into New York City's busiest emergency room, where I worked.

Shortly after I started working in the E.R., a young teenage boy came for a checkup. People did that sometimes back then — used the E.R. as a doctor's office. He looked healthy, but said he had been feeling a little off and thought he might have a cold or the flu. The doctor examined him but didn't see anything wrong. "All right," he told the young man, "you look fine. You're probably just working out too much. But let's be sure. We'll draw some blood to check for white cells, see if there's an infection.

And we'll take a urine sample."

I gave the boy a few minutes alone, then went back and took the little cup he handed me. As I left the examining room, I looked down and saw that his urine had a green hue.

I hurried to the doctor and showed him the urine sample. He looked at it, then glanced at me with a slight frown.

"It's so awful that he has leukemia," I said with compassion. I assumed the doctor, too, saw what had struck me as an unmistakable sign of the disease.

The doctor, however, had seen nothing of the sort. He thought I was nuts – until the lab results came back showing the markers for leukemia. Then he thought I was scary.

Although this kind of sudden "knowing" happened more and more often in my work as a trauma/E.R. nurse, it didn't put a dent in my denial that I was an intuitive. After all, there was no such thing.

Ironically though, the more I doubted the veracity of my gift, the stronger became the evidence for it. No matter how hard I worked at ignoring or finding logical explanations for the phenomena I was experiencing, one thing became perfectly clear. Before the lab tests were run, I knew my patient's diagnosis.

When a woman came in with abdominal pain, I knew whether it was appendicitis, an ectopic pregnancy, an ovarian cyst, or one of the six or seven other diagnoses that fit her symptoms. With one look, I knew when heart patients were about to go into cardiac arrest. The fact that I had an uncanny – and uncannily accurate – sixth sense was lost on me though. I simply thought I was a great E.R. nurse and that, like all E.R. nurses, I was operating from gut instinct. I didn't realize that my "gut instinct" was profoundly more developed than that of my colleagues.

One afternoon, a slightly overweight man in his late fifties named Jon came into the E.R. complaining of indigestion. Naturally, the staff went into overdrive because he was the right age and weight to be at high risk for a heart attack. We did an immediate EKG, ran some blood tests, and hooked him up to a cardiac monitor.

All of Jon's tests came out normal, and I didn't pick up any hidden arterial blockage that could lead to a heart attack. So we asked what he had for lunch. It was pepperoni pizza. Well, we thought, who hasn't gotten indigestion from a pepperoni pizza? We gave him some Maalox and his indigestion went away. Just to be on the safe side, though, Jon was sent up to the cardiac monitoring floor for twenty-four hours.

The next morning he was released, and he stopped by to thank me for my nursing care. On the outside Jon looked great. But something was nagging at me, distracting me from our conversation. My internal alarms were clanging, but I didn't exactly know why.

Jon must have sensed I was distracted, because he cut the conversation short and said goodbye. As he walked out of the E.R. and the automatic door whooshed shut behind him, I had a brief and terrible vision. Jon was lying face down with his cheek on the pavement. A small abrasion marked his forehead, and he had no heartbeat. I couldn't tell if this was going to happen in the next moment or in the next year, but it was clear Jon was going to die. Then I realized that in the vision, Jon was wearing the same clothes he had on today. I sprinted out the door yelling for him.

It was like being in a slow-motion dream. Jon turned, recognized me, and smiled. Then it was as if the switch sending current to his heart had been suddenly flipped off. He dropped face down on the pavement and was dead before he hit the ground. I shouted for help, knelt beside him, and turned him on his back. Just before I thumped him directly on his sternum, I noticed an abrasion on his forehead from where it had hit the sidewalk.

The force of the blow was enough to restart Jon's heart. He was rushed back into the E.R. and eventually wheeled into surgery to get an automatic defibrillator implanted.

Jon had suffered sudden adult death syndrome, which can happen to very healthy-looking people. Sometimes, for no apparent reason – no blockage, no history of heart disease – the heart begins to beat rapidly and erratically. Then the electrical system of the heart suddenly fails. Nothing signals the heart to beat, and it stops pumping blood. This is called ventricular fibrillation. If you are lucky enough to have a trained professional at hand who can thump your chest (this resets the heart's electrical system) or be near a defibrillator that can give your heart a jolt of electricity, you will survive. If not, you will die.

Of all the technical and emotional skills I had to learn as a trauma nurse, the hardest to master was accepting the fact that I was intuitive. However, once I stopped fighting it and shifted from my old stance as the New York skeptic who says "Absolutely not!" to a new – but still cautious – stance of intellectual curiosity, the E.R. became a whole new kind of training ground for me.

I started to learn how different diseases "look" psychically. I became skilled at distinguishing the **energetic signature** of cancer from that of AIDS or multiple sclerosis. I learned that the signature of chronic fatigue is similar to that of fibromyalgia.

I also learned that when a person is only a few hours away from death, his energy field, instead of radiating out from his body, looks like a white cloud hanging a few feet above it. When a person is ready to die, this cloud turns a dense grayish-black and rises to the ceiling. The process is gradual and, depending on the circumstances, can take several minutes to a few days. One day a woman called the emergency room needing to know how badly her son had been hurt in a car accident. I looked at him and saw that his energy field was about two feet above his body. I knew this meant he had only hours to live, so I told her to come to the hospital without delay. Ninety minutes later, I saw that his essence had floated up near the ceiling. I knew he had broken the bonds with his body and wasn't coming back. He died within the hour, his mother at his side.

Energetic Signature

The unique electromagnetic vibration that emanates from each living thing. This vibration can be detected by certain people or by use of a spectroscopic microscope. The energetic signature serves as a unique identifier for every single being or substance that exists. Even identical twins have different energetic signatures.

When someone died in the E.R. and we were able to bring him back to life, I could also see the energy return to the body. I learned over time that when a person's essence is just above his body, it sometimes means that he is deciding whether or not to leave this life. I saw this with terminally ill patients a lot. When I would check back in about an hour, the patient's energy would either have dropped closer to his body – signaling that he had chosen to stay a while longer – or have risen even further – because he was getting ready to leave for good.

Having this special knowledge taught me that I was different from other nurses in the E.R. My knowing when someone was about to go into cardiac arrest often confounded my co-workers. While it was a good thing for the patient, it scared the other nurses. One woman told me she was afraid I would see something bad about her; others believed that my seeing something bad about them could create that reality. I had a gift that many people regarded as a curse or a form of madness. Others denied it even existed – there was certainly no listing for Medical Intuitives in the Yellow Pages.

At this point, I needed to make a choice: I could be open and willing to receive all that came with my gift (including things that were painful to know, like seeing that the young man had leukemia) and act on what I saw, or I could worry about looking like an idiot and keep my mouth closed.

I was pushed into making a decision the following Tuesday. It was one of those nights where the hands on the clock don't budge, the patients don't move upstairs to their assigned beds, and the thought of scrubbing your bathroom seems more appealing and interesting than what you're doing right now. Then all hell broke loose.

There had been a terrible auto accident. My patient was fourteen and his body had been badly mangled. His ribs were crushed. His left lung had collapsed. Blood had collected in the pericardial sac around his heart, creating a compression of the heart that would soon cause cardiac standstill. There was blood everywhere, IVs were sprouting from both his arms. When we tapped into his belly with a catheter to check for internal bleeding, blood spurted to the ceiling. We tried everything. We put in chest tubes to inflate the lung, administered drugs to boost the heart beat, inserted tubes for breathing.

But it was a losing battle from the start, and it didn't take my gift to figure that out. He died in the E.R., and I said a prayer for the boy and his family, deeply saddened by the loss of such a young life.

While I waited for the boy's family to arrive, Father Mark arrived to give him last rites. Father Mark was a fixture in the E.R. We saw him often – all too often, considering his sad purpose – yet he rarely acknowledged any of us beyond a nod of greeting or the question "Which room?" We admired his strength, as he often witnessed gruesome, bloody, and fatal injuries but never wavered in his duties, never vomited, and never looked away as so many non-medical personnel did.

When I saw Father Mark headed for the dead boy's room, something told me to intercept him. I knew better than to question it. I grabbed his arm and motioned him into the quiet room.

"This is really a tough one, Father Mark. It will be very hard to see."

"It's always hard," he replied briskly. "Excuse me. I have to go administer last rites." He started back toward the boy's room.

Again something nagged at me. For some reason, I didn't want him to go into that room. "Father Mark," I said, "let's call another priest. This one isn't for you."

He looked at me with both surprise and consternation. "Look, you know I've been around bad traumas and shootings, young and old. It's just a person's shell in that room, his soul is gone," he said. "I've done this before, you know."

I nodded, surprised at the edge to his voice. Still, I couldn't let him go. I was overcome with a deep, deep sorrow. I didn't understand what was happening, but this time I didn't waste time questioning myself.

I rested my hand on Father Mark's forearm and said, "I'd like to prepare you for what you're going to see." Then I described the scene that awaited him. I knew I needed to be explicit and not sugarcoat anything. When I was done, I walked with him into the room.

"I am staying with you," I announced. He seemed surprised, but went ahead and gave the boy last rites.

When we left the room, Father Mark was quite pale and shaky. I walked him back to the quiet room. Tears were rolling down his cheeks.

"Thank you," he said in a stricken voice. "That was the nicest thing anyone has ever done for me in a hospital. Your compassion will never be forgotten."

I didn't understand what Father Mark meant until I received a note from him several days later. He wrote that he had lost his fifteen-year-old brother in a similar auto accident. Father Mark was just eighteen at the time, but the E.R. nurses let him walk into his brother's room without any explanation or preparation for the terrible sight he would see. The sight of his beloved little brother mangled and bloody had scarred him deeply. He carried anger at those nurses for thirty years.

Reading that note, I knew my decision had been made. I would open fully to my gift and act on the knowledge I received without fear of what others would think.

Once I accepted my intuition, other people began to accept it too. Some of the nurses would quietly ask me about their families or a particular patient. Sometimes they'd ask about their love lives, promotions, or which horse would win at the track.

Because I had lost my fear and begun to respect my gift, others did too. Gradually the questions about the horses ceased. Although I was glad to no longer be regarded as a freak, my experience with Father Mark taught me that others' opinions of my gift didn't matter. It came down to this: I had a choice to focus my gift on life, joy, God, happiness, and health, or worry about my reputation. The choice was simple – and it determined my destiny.

CHAPTER 3

The Failure of 'Recipe Medicine'

As the distinguished physicist Henri Poincaré once said,
"It is through science that we prove, but
through intuition that we discover."

Revealing my profession brings varied responses. Sometimes I hear, "Oh, how fascinating to see the future." And in the next breath, "What do you see about *me?*" Others are less self-absorbed. They simply look askance at me, nod silently to themselves – and move far, far away.

I remember being at an elegant cocktail party replete with physicians and researchers in the field of cancer. It was hosted by one of our patients, and I was invited because I was part of her health care team. Treading cautiously, I spoke about the invisible but very real energetics of illness, which I'll explain in the next chapter.

For some reason, my information greatly threatened those of the old school of medicine. There was not an iota of openness, curiosity, or willingness to hear more. Their shut-down body language and disapproving facial expressions could have been seen a mile away. Even though I had a second-degree black belt in karate, I never instilled such fear as I did that night. The dividing line at the party was evident. After my little talk, I looked up to find the Western-medicine practitioners on one side of the room ... and me on the other.

Despite having worked with cancer patients for quite a while and being part of that health care team (I was the token complementary-medicine practitioner), that night I suddenly became a threatening and strange creature because I spoke up about what I do. It broke the unwritten "Don't ask, don't tell" pact that apparently many of my colleagues thought they had with me. (Even now, doctors often say to my clients, "I don't want to know what you're doing with her, but keep doing it. You're looking good!")

I was saddened by their fear, that night and in the years since. A good Medical Intuitive can be invaluable on a health care team, often picking up a problem that Western medicine has overlooked.

Ironically, intuition is – and always has been – an important part of medical practice, whether conventional or alternative. Fifty years ago, when doctors still made house calls, family physicians used their education, their experience, *and* their intuition to diagnose whether grandmother's chest pain was angina, heartburn, or deep grief for grandfather, who'd passed away the month before. Now we are so in awe of the scientific advances in Western medicine, we rely solely on technology to tell us what a patient's problem is.

The same is happening in complementary medicine. Traditionally, an acupuncturist made his diagnosis intuitively. Then he would confirm it by checking the nature of the patient's pulses (there are twenty-eight different kinds of pulses described in Traditional Chinese Medicine). Today, unfortunately, most of the acupuncture schools in the United States teach students to make their diagnosis predominantly by reading the pulses.

When did this fear of intuition take hold? When did we begin the transition to what I call "recipe medicine," the practice in conventional medicine of exclusively following a prescribed formula to diagnose and treat illness? Such a practice can make a doctor lax, as it often results in her not fully hearing or seeing her patients.

Energy Field

The area around the human body into which the electromagnetic energy that the cells of our bodies naturally produce is projected. The energy in this field vibrates at frequencies that change depending on your physical health and well-being. When you are healthy, the energy in this field vibrates at a high frequency. When you are unwell, it vibrates at a low frequency. Your energy field is also called your aura or etheric field.

Sadly, complementary medicine has followed suit. Books abound attesting to the "energetic profile" of someone with pain in the hip (he has "a fear of moving forward") or chronic fatigue (he is rooted in the belief that he's "not good enough"). I am grateful to the pioneers in this field, but I don't believe they meant for us to follow a recipe and discard our intuition. This can too easily lead to an inaccurate diagnosis – which means continued pain and suffering for the patient.

For example, I recently scanned the **energy field** of a woman who afterwards took me to task for not identifying her predominant illness. Rhonda told me she had rheumatoid arthritis and had long suffered from disabling pain and stiffness. I told her that I hadn't seen any sign of rheumatoid arthritis in her. She assured me that her blood tests had come back positive for the illness and several rheumatologists had confirmed the diagnosis.

As further proof, Rhonda said, she matched the "energetic profile" for rheumatoid arthritis. An alternative-medicine practitioner told her that the origin of her illness was that she felt "very put upon." Upon hearing this, Rhonda acknowledged that her ex-husband had dominated her and routinely violated her personal boundaries.

Unfortunately, before being examined, Rhonda told the alternative-medicine practitioner that she had been diagnosed with rheumatoid arthritis. My guess is that he simply looked up the supposed "energetic profile" for that illness and told her what it was.

What I saw when I scanned Rhonda's physical body and her energy field was not that she felt put upon, but that she had a pattern of distancing herself from God (which is how she thought of her Higher Power) and from any man who cared for her. She originally stopped going to church because she was angry at God for the suffering she was going through in her marriage. Rhonda hated her ex-husband and lived in dread of being punished by God for these feelings. For her, it was wrong to hate. She thought she just should have tried harder to be a good wife.

Rhonda continued to argue with me about the "fact" that she had rheumatoid arthritis until finally I apologized — with some vehemence — that she did *not* have rheumatoid arthritis, but had the parvovirus instead. That's what was causing the pain in her joints.

Fortunately, Rhonda wanted to be well more than she wanted to be right. She returned to her physician and chose her words cautiously. She asked if there could be any unusual cause for her arthritis. After some speculation, he considered the idea of a virus. She requested that he humor her and test for it. The test was positive, Rhonda began treatment for the parvovirus, and within seven weeks she was a new and very happy woman.

This case gives you a good example of how I work. It shows the ideal situation, where my medical intuition and the wonders of modern medical science collaborate in the best interests of the patient. I don't scoff at Western medicine. I spent too many years working as a registered nurse in some of New York and New Jersey's busiest and best emergency rooms and trauma centers. I know firsthand what the wonder of modern science can do for people in pain.

I also know what it can't do.

CHAPTER 4

It's All About Energy

*Our health and our happiness depend entirely
on the amount of energy flowing through us.*

A ll physical illness begins in your energy system. Let me explain what I mean. For nearly a century, starting with Einstein, scientists have known that what Hamlet called his "too too solid flesh" only *seems* solid because we can only perceive it with our five senses. When looked at through a stronger lens – the perspective of quantum physics – we are a collection of constantly moving molecules, atoms, and subatomic particles: in other words, pure energy.

You don't have to depend on science to grasp this concept, though. Simple common sense tells you that illness begins in your **energy system**.

At one time or another, you have no doubt had the experience of letting yourself get run down and catching the cold or flu that is going around. You know that getting run down – whether because of prolonged lack of sleep, overwork, or emotional distress – lowers your resistance to illness. Every part of you gets sluggish, from your muscles to your immune system to your mind. Getting out of bed feels like a Herculean task. Making decisions is impossible. Your energy level is just too low.

.Energy is your basic life force. You can *feel* it in yourself. We have all had days when we felt happy and full of energy, or sad and depleted. Our energy level increases or decreases when there are positive or negative changes in our lives, whether they be changes in the body, mind, heart, or spirit. Even been brokenhearted? Betrayed by someone you love? Depressed or lonely? Then you know that when you feel low emotionally, your health declines too. You literally don't have the energy to fight off illness.

For now, though, let's focus on the energy of the body. I'll talk more about the mind – and the heart – in the next chapter.

All living things, from plankton to presidents, emit electromagnetic energy. This energy, which is present in every cell in the body, radiates from us in the form of vibrations.

These electromagnetic vibrations can be read and measured by diagnostic instruments as common nowadays as CAT scans and MRI scanners. The results of these read-

Energy System

The human energy system has two parts: the electromagnetic energy field, which is located outside the body, and the seven major energy centers within the body.

These seven energy centers are called **chakras**. They are located near your spine, and run from the top of your head (the "crown" chakra) to your tailbone (the "root" chakra). Each correlates to major clusters of nerve cells (called ganglia) that branch out from your spinal cord.

The chakras also correlate to different physical and emotional energies. I'll talk more about this in the chapters to come.

ings are interpreted by experienced professionals who can diagnose whether the patient has a heart irregularity, a brain tumor, or nothing whatsoever wrong with him.

As a Medical Intuitive, I do the same thing, only on a broader level. I read and measure your energy by scanning your entire body – not just a specific area like your heart or brain, as an MRI or a CAT scan would do. At the same time, I also scan your energy field, reading the electromagnetic vibration in the area immediately outside your body. Like the people who read and interpret MRIs, I am an experienced medical professional. I can identify not only the frequency (ranging from high to low) of the vibration in your chakras and energy field, but what disease – if any – it indicates.

While each disease has its own unique frequency, all diseases have a low vibration. This is another reason why a Medical Intuitive can pick up signs of illness that modern medicine cannot. Besides scanning the whole body, not just the area where the symptoms have appeared, I can sense vibrations across a much broader range of frequencies than today's medical equipment can register.

How can a human being possibly pick up signs of illness that our most sophisticated medical equipment cannot? Like the statement I opened this chapter with – "All physical illness begins in your energy system" – it only sounds odd because you haven't stopped to think about it.

To start with, we know that certain people can perceive things in ways that science has not yet been able to explain. We have all heard stories of people who *knew* when a loved one was in danger or had suddenly died. Perhaps you have had this happen yourself. We don't scoff at these kinds of experiences anymore. They have too often proved true.

This is now an accepted part of our understanding of how

the world works. We don't care that it is supposedly impossible for people to know such things about distant loved ones. We know it happens. We no longer doubt that sometimes human beings are able to communicate nonverbally over great distances. Through some mechanism we don't yet understand, our human sensing "equipment" is extremely sensitive to sudden declines in the energetic vibration of special people in our lives. In fact, our inborn vibration-sensors are far more sensitive than anything science has yet developed.

Physical Ways to Raise Your Vibration...

◆ Have great sex.
◆ Play sports you love.
◆ Get plenty of sleep.
◆ Dance!
◆ Eat healthy *and* delicious foods.
◆ Play with your pet.

...or Lower It

◆ Watch TV instead of making love.
◆ Never get out-of-doors.
◆ Eat mostly fast food.
◆ Sleep as little as possible.
◆ Never move your body just for the pleasure of it.
◆ Drink heavily or smoke at least a half a pack a day.
◆ Take "recreational" drugs.

The ability to perceive the energetic vibration of other people is like any other human ability, from singing to sprinting. If you work on developing it, you get better at it. This is why I can read and analyze others' energetic vibration. I may have been born with a heightened sensitivity to others' energy – just as some people are born with perfect pitch – but I have also been honing my gift for more than fifteen years. Why do you need to know about high-frequency and low-frequency vibration? Two reasons. First, because you have the ability to either **raise or lower your vibration**, which has a direct impact on your health and happiness. Second, because in the world of vibrations, like attracts like, and you want to be very careful of what vibrations you invite in. Low vibrations attract other low vibrations.

High vibrations **resonate** with other high vibrations.

This law of vibrational attraction is another experience we have all had. Think back to a time when you met someone with whom you immediately "clicked." You sensed in her a like-minded person, someone who would "get" you. Communicating with her was a snap. Sometimes you didn't even need words. A look would do it. A shrug of the shoulders. You were operating on the same wave length.

Well, that was literally true. The frequency of your electromagnetic vibration – high, low, or in between – was in synch with the other person's. You resonated with each other.

The same thing happens

Resonate

In the language of energy medicine, to resonate means to have energy that is vibrating at the same frequency as something else. It's like in a music store, when you pluck the G string on a guitar. Suddenly all the G strings on the other guitars begin to vibrate too. They are resonating with the frequency of the first string, responding to its vibration with an identical vibration of their own.

In very simple terms, this is how your body and psyche attract illness: When your vibration drops, whether for physical or emotional reasons, you resonate with the low vibration of illness.

with illness. When your energy drops from the high vibration of good health to the low vibration of exhaustion or depression, you risk resonating with the low vibration of heart disease, cancer, diabetes, or the common cold. This is how you "catch" a disease.

Now, we don't usually talk about "catching" cancer or heart disease, but this is actually what happens (unless the illness, like some types of cancer, is caused by environmental toxins like asbestos or radioactivity.) When your energy vibrates at the same low frequency as a particular illness, you are opening a direct line to it, so to speak. And the longer your vibration continues to be low, the greater risk you run for contracting the illness.

This is what is so helpful about medical intuition. Because all illness begins in your energy system, a Medical Intuitive can detect a low vibration in your energy field and chakras before a full-blown illness takes hold.

We're like an elegant early-warning system, the best kind of preventive medicine.

Now You Know...

◆ All illness begins in your energy system. PAGE 27.

◆ Your energy is manifested in an electromagnetic vibration within and just beyond the physical limits of your
body. PAGE 28.

◆ The frequency of this vibration increases or decreases
depending on your health and well-being. PAGE 30.

◆ All diseases have a low vibration. PAGE 29.

◆ Because like attracts like, if your energy is consistently
at a low vibration, it will attract illness. When this happens, we say you "resonate" with the illness. PAGE 31.

◆ Medical intuition is the best preventive medicine because it detects a low vibration in your energy system
before the illness invades your actual body. PAGE 32.

CHAPTER 5

Face to Face With My Worst Fear

Be careful what you ask for. You just might get it.

Even after my experience with Father Mark and my decision to embrace my gift, at times it was more than I bargained for. It was heartbreaking and frustrating when I could see a patient's outcome or diagnosis but knew that in his case, there was nothing I could do to change it. His disease had progressed too far, or his soul had decided it was time for him to go.

Then there would be days when my intuition was a godsend. This was especially true in deciding how to handle new admissions to the E.R. There were never enough nurses to go around, and the nursing staff could get stretched dangerously thin — emotionally as well as physically — if we tried to care for everyone at once. Thanks to my sixth sense, I could tell whether a new patient's condition was life-threatening or not, even before we did a workup on her. This allowed me to focus my efforts on the seriously ill and wounded, and worry less about making the others wait a little longer.

As helpful as my gift was at times, it was still scary for others. If I accidentally made an intuitive diagnosis aloud, some of my fellow trauma nurses would pull away from me as though I had the evil eye. I suppose it must have been frightening to hear me say I had to stay with a certain patient because she was getting worse, when to all appearances she looked completely stable. It must have been even worse when that patient suddenly went into crisis. They struggled with being loyal to their beliefs that psychic gifts were phony, or accepting that my premonitions came true.

Just as it seemed that I had gotten comfortable with my intuition, a new aspect of my gift would emerge. I had no intuition teacher, curriculum, or control over which gifts would emerge when. I knew I needed more help than this world could give, so I prayed for divine **guidance**.

In the beginning – like many people – I couldn't discern whether what came to me was divine guidance or my own thoughts. Now I know that my confusion stemmed from the fact that I was so busy telling God exactly what kind of divine guidance I wanted, I couldn't hear anything else. My demands were:

- Don't let people think I'm a nut.

- Only tell me things I want to hear.

- Tell me everything I need to do and tell me now. I don't want to hear it bit by bit over time.

- Give me a complete

Guidance

Advice and instructions that come to you from God (or your Higher Power, the Divine, the Self, Spirit, or whatever term you use for the universal loving presence available to us all). Your guidance will always point you in the direction of your greatest good because God is the source of the highest vibration of all: unconditional love.

outline of how to use my gift, including concrete, logistical information.

Eventually I would have to face several important – and uncomfortable – truths about guidance. First, praying for guidance requires that you be fully open to whatever answer comes. You can't put conditions on the guidance you ask for. For example, I prayed for guidance on how to use my intuitive gift, but my mind wasn't quiet and open. I only wanted to hear one thing: Continue to do the nursing work you love, and just use your intuition when it's needed.

That's *not* what I heard. This taught me the second important truth about guidance: You will not always like the guidance you receive. I certainly didn't.

What was this unwelcome guidance? To use my remaining time in the E.R. – it wasn't clear how long that would be – to refine my intuitive gift and conquer my biggest fear: death.

"Hey, that's not the answer to my prayers!" I protested.

But God knew better, and that was the answer I got.

You probably find it strange that I worked in a trauma center when my biggest fear was death. Why would I choose to spend eight to sixteen hours a day in a place where people often died bloody and painful deaths? For the same reason the chicken crossed the road: to get to the other side. In my case, it was to get to the other side of my fear. Besides, working in the E.R. hadn't been something I thought up, remember? God had put me exactly where I needed to be to face my demons.

Like most deep fears, mine began in childhood. During a period of about five years, starting when I was in first grade, death took four important people from my life without warning. The first was my beloved grandfather, who died unexpectedly when I was seven. Next was my neighbor and buddy "Mr. Oatmeal," whose sudden death I foresaw when I was eight. Then another neighbor, a young, healthy, and apparently happy woman who was like a second mother to me, put a gun to her head one day and pulled the trigger. Out of the blue. No one knew she had been feeling suicidal. The fourth was a girl my own age, an elementary school playmate, who collapsed and died without warning, a victim of what we now know as sudden death syndrome.

From a child's point of view, people are not supposed to die suddenly – and certainly not young. Severe car crashes were understandable, and old age, but what did it mean when my "other mom" and my playmate died suddenly? To me, it meant that the world was not safe. You could lose a parent or friend in an instant. It meant that the world was not logical or orderly – these weren't old people dying of old age. Worst of all, it meant that I was mortal, and one day I would die too. This was too much for my young mind to handle. It made me so afraid that I couldn't look at a dead body at a wake. I was inconsolable at funerals. Death was scarier than the boogeyman in my closet.

My fear was intensified by the culture I grew up in. As a Catholic child of the sixties, I learned that people who didn't confess their sins and get absolution would burn in hell. I figured that had to include everyone who died suddenly, since they didn't have time for confession and absolution. I was horrified to think that my buddy Mr. Oatmeal must have gone straight to hell.

I had also learned that even if you did confess your sins and get absolution, as my grandfather had, you went to purgatory, where you were punished and purified by fire until you were in a fit state to ascend to heaven. I had recurring nightmares of Grandpa clinging to a long, long ladder while flames blistered the soles of his feet.

God had put me in the E.R. to help me face my fear of

death, which was rooted in these sudden losses and my fear of purgatory. I would like to report that my nurse's training eased my fears, but it didn't. As a medical professional, I was able to save some lives and help prepare others for the death of their bodies, but what about their souls? The end of life was still a frightening mystery to me. What happened to our souls after death? Did they die too, or did some part of us continue somehow? Would they get absorbed in the ether and just disappear? Would I end up on that fiery ladder next to Granddad, howling in pain?

I needed answers, and I thought I was ready to heal my fear of death. For the second time, I prayed for divine guidance. This time, I learned two lessons about prayer. First, our Higher Power will never fail to answer us when we ask. Second, don't ask for something until you are truly ready to get it!

I had no idea that the events of that lovely spring day would so fully answer my prayers, or that God's answer would look so different from mine. It started with a feeling that something strange was going to happen; it was as if my angels were giving me a heads-up that I would be learning something new. The impression I got was, "Buckle up! This could be a bumpy ride!"

Early in the afternoon, a cheerful young man of twenty named Jeff came in to the E.R. While working as a tree cutter, he had fallen from a limb and landed – hard – right on his head. Jeff had not lost consciousness, though, and he said he felt fine. His boss insisted he come in and get checked out anyway. There was not a scratch, bruise, or bump on Jeff's head. Yet looking at him, I heard my guidance tell me that Jeff would die shortly. *Stay with him*, it added.

All my old fears of death came flooding back. I was now a fully trained and more than competent E.R. nurse, but this vibrant young man without a mark on him was still going to die.

My Catholic faith said that if he died without confessing his sins, he would go to hell. If he did confess, he'd go to purgatory – still a scary place. If this wasn't bad enough, I was no longer completely convinced by the dogma of my church, so maybe Jeff would just become food for the worms. Maybe this life was all there was – and his was so short.

A CAT scan of Jeff's head was done, and I stayed with him while we waited for the results. I prayed, but I knew I could not change the outcome. My guidance again was clear: *Stay with him when he leaves his body. Stay with him when he crosses over.*

My feelings went from anger at this young man's too-early death to shock and fear at the thought of crossing over with him. I nearly fainted. Over *there* was the last place I wanted to go. The image of my grandfather standing on that ladder with burned feet was still with me. I was supposed to go *there*? The idea was not frightening, it was galling! Here I was in the business of saving people's lives – and my guidance was telling me to get in the cosmic car with Jeff and drop him off in purgatory?

The next moment another thought hit me like a lightning bolt: *What if I can't get back?* I nearly burst into tears. I desperately wanted to run from the room. Probably the only thing that kept me there was that I have some sort of "nurse gene." I couldn't let Jeff go to his death alone – I couldn't think of anything scarier. I wasn't going to allow it to happen.

As the minutes wore on, Jeff became increasingly quiet. Gradually his conversation and laughter stopped altogether. He slowly curled up into the fetal position and closed his eyes. Then I saw a sort of white light start to rise from his body. By the time his CAT scan results came back, Jeff had made his last sounds. His brain stem had been sheared by the impact of his fall. There is no treatment for that.

The doctor came in and shrugged. He left, closing the door

behind him. I laid my hand protectively on Jeff's upper arm and spoke softly to him about God's love for us, but I felt like a fraud. How could a loving God send people to suffer in purgatory? Jeff was now unconscious, but hearing is the last sense to go, so I told him simply that I would stay with him and he wouldn't die alone.

Saying that Jeff didn't die alone is an understatement.

One minute I could hear the busy E.R., the pounding of my frightened heart and Jeff's ever-slowing breath, and the next minute I saw Jeff's spirit completely lift from his body and hover in the room. I was too shocked to react. My human brain could not comprehend what was happening. Then I felt myself lift up and out of my own body. I was hovering with Jeff, feeling his pain and shock – then suddenly feeling his awe as all earthly suffering fell away. How can I describe the experience of losing one's physical form and becoming pure spirit? What words can express floating in a bright, sweetly scented place without boundaries?

A multitude of thoughts raced through my mind: *Am I dead? This feels good! Hey, it's very light in here.* I was awestruck as I looked down and saw our physical selves in the hospital room.

And that's when it happened. That's when I learned that all I had been taught was false. There is no pain or suffering after death. I was in the outskirts of the most beautiful place imaginable. I was overwhelmed with the immensity of God's huge and unconditional love. I floated at the edges of the brightest light and breathed in a joy unknown in this world. And I was only standing on the threshold. Suddenly I realized that Jeff was no longer with me. He had crossed that threshold and gone inside. His physical outline shimmered and gradually faded from my view. He had become indistinguishable from the love and joy surrounding him. It felt like I stood there watching him for an eternity, and I yearned to follow him. I realized I was happy for

Jeff. Happy that he had died.

At that moment I knew I would never fear death again. I understood that **crossing over** was not a terrible thing after all. After death there is no pain, no anger, no jealousy – only light and joy and the knowledge that you will never be alone again.

I thought of all the people I knew who had died, and I was suddenly at peace. I had experienced the difference between living on earth in a physical body and being set free. Earth seemed so dense and dark and smelly and loud compared to this place.

Then I felt myself falling backward. I was in the examination room again, back in my body. Looking at Jeff's lifeless body on the gurney, I was speechless with wonder. I had experienced firsthand the difference between the soul and the body, and knew that purgatory was bogus. I felt like I had gone home.

I was shown that death is not to be feared. It is merely a transition into a different form, an ethereal form. I learned that your body dies, but your essence continues. Most important, I learned that you are not alone in the moment of death. When you cross over you are met by pure love. You can call this place heaven if you want or you can simply think of it as a place of very, very high vibration. Either way, it is the greatest experience you will ever have.

Crossing Over

When your soul leaves your physical body, usually at death, and goes to a place of pure love and pure spirit, which many call heaven.

Jeff's leaving that night was both terrible and beautiful. After returning to my body, my human self cried for Jeff, for the tragedy of his dying so young, never having experienced marriage or fatherhood, or achieving the wisdom that only comes with age. I think I cried for myself, too. A huge weight had been lifted; my worst fear had been healed. A sense of joy and longing filled me.

To this day, I continue to cross over with people. If they know they are going to die and are very frightened, I sometimes show them where they are going to go ahead of time.

I still don't know what to call this place. But I do know that our spirit doesn't die when our physical body does.

Now You Know...

◆ When you ask for divine guidance, you have to be open to whatever answer comes. PAGE 37.

◆ You will not always like the guidance you receive! PAGE 37.

◆ Your Higher Power will never fail to help you when you ask, so don't ask for something until you are ready to receive it. PAGE 39.

◆ After death there is no pain, no anger, no jealousy — only light and joy and the knowledge that you will never be alone again. PAGE 41.

CHAPTER 6

The Power of Your Thoughts and Feelings

Here's the good news: Your body believes
exactly what you believe. That's also the bad news.

The people who consult me for medical reasons are either ill
and know it, or they just don't feel right. In either case,
they can identify their symptoms, but they (and often their doctors) don't know what's really wrong.

This is one of the advantages of consulting a Medical Intuitive. I don't look at symptoms. Symptoms can be misleading. I
look directly at what's *causing* those symptoms. I do this by scanning your energy field and your seven energy centers. When a
diagnosis is based on energy, it can be trusted. Energy never lies.

A person's energy field, for example, has a distinct look
when he is near death. In the E.R., I cared for many heart attack
patients with hard-driving Type A personalities, who, according

to medical standards, were stable. Their vital signs were good, their color was great, they had steady heart beats and were free of chest pain. It was disconcerting to watch their energy fields gradually fade from a translucent white to a dense grayish black. Within the hour, these patients would go into cardiac arrest and die.

At times like these, I felt profoundly inadequate as a health care provider. Either we had missed the real cause of these people's illness, or we were only treating the symptoms, which meant that the person would feel better for a while – until the untreated underlying illness caused new symptoms, that is. Then, more than likely, we would see them back in the E.R. again.

Why didn't we look at the cause and begin there? My ongoing frustration and regret pushed me to explore ways to use my intuitive abilities to help people truly heal. What I discovered both surprised me and made perfect sense.

In the E.R. there generally wasn't much room for old-fashioned, compassionate bedside nursing. Our waiting room was packed, and there was just enough time to stabilize a patient before having to move on to the next. Sometimes, however, I got the rare opportunity to sit with a patient. This was the case with a young woman named Dora.

Dora was a vibrant, chatty twenty-three-year-old who reported having had cramping in her lower stomach for two days. She wasn't pregnant, didn't have giardia, and had no fever, nausea, or diarrhea. Nor was her pain – which was severe – localized in the right lower quadrant, which would have been a pretty sure sign she had appendicitis. Instead, Dora's symptoms pointed to a diagnosis of stress.

I disagreed. What I saw when I read Dora was acute appendicitis. Her appendix itself "looked" dark, contracted, and in-

flamed. Her vibration was also low, which is indicative of inflammation. Appendicitis can be very serious if not treated immediately. When the appendix gets inflamed, it can rupture,
spew infection into the abdominal cavity, and cause death.

The standard procedure for someone with Dora's symptoms
was to draw blood in order to check her white blood cell count
and to take abdominal x-rays. The doctor ordered the tests, even
though she didn't think they would show anything.

I went ahead and drew Dora's blood, however, and as I did I
saw a swirling mass of energy around her head. I picked up the
vibration of confusion and chaos, though she was talking to me
quite normally. Though my conscious mind already knew her diagnosis, I found my eyes unconsciously scanning her chakras. In
her root chakra at the base of her torso, I saw what looked like a
black hole. The root chakra is the energy center for our survival
instincts. Blackness in any chakra means the chakra has become
blocked, and the person has no energy for that area of her life. In
this case, since the blackness was in the root, or first chakra, it
meant that Dora feared for her survival.

In my mind's eye I suddenly saw an image of a man hovering
next to Dora. He was clearly someone with whom she was involved. I heard screaming and fighting, and saw an image of Dora
immobilized by her fear of being hurt and too terrified to get out
of the relationship. She was on the verge of being physically
abused but couldn't save herself.

As the scene unfolded, I put my hands on Dora's head. I
could feel her unrelenting thoughts ricocheting around her brain
like a ping pong ball. She had become completely helpless, unable to think straight or make decisions. The chaos swirling
around her head had increased dramatically. Normally there are
calm waves of energy around a person – like the gentle ripples in
a pond after a small stone is tossed in it. In Dora's case, it was as

if someone had heaved a boulder in that pond, causing a near tidal wave.

When the scene faded, I realized Dora had stopped talking and was looking at me with an open and trusting gaze.

"You know, don't you?" she whispered.

I nodded. "Has he hit you?" I inquired gently.

"Not yet," she said, looking down in shame. "Not yet."

I squeezed her hand. "We need to have a chat." I told her that her appendix needed to come out, and that living in this state of chaos had contributed to her condition. I told her this was a wakeup call, and that there were people who could and would help her out of her frightening situation.

"But it has to be your choice," I said. "Only you can make this choice." We talked briefly, and Dora said she would do whatever it took to change her life.

I went and told the E.R. doctor that my gut feeling was that we should keep Dora overnight for observation. Although Dora's test results were back – her white count was normal and her x-rays were negative – the doctor trusted my instinct. The next day, Dora's appendix was taken out, and social services began helping her get out of her dangerous relationship and start over.

After my experience with Dora, I began taking note of my patients' personality traits and any significant events they chose to share with me. While I did not read anyone without his or her permission, I did note each person's energy field – and found significant similarities. For example, patients with multiple sclerosis had the same energetic pattern. Every depressed patient had a thin, gray, and hazy energy field, but there were subtle differences between medically diagnosable, chronic depression and a short-term depression brought on by the loss of a loved one or other painful event.

At this time, I started doing "unofficial" readings outside the

E.R. when friends or family asked me to, and I began to see in these people's energy fields the same kind of thing I saw in Dora's: Their negative emotions, thoughts, and unhealthy patterns of behavior were lowering their vibrations and allowing illness to resonate with their bodies. I understood that simply treating the symptoms would not raise a person's vibration, it would merely buy time. In Dora's case, removing her appendix was palliative but necessary medicine. The organ was inflamed and therefore removed. Had she not cleaned up the abuse issue, her vibration would have remained low and she would have resonated with another health problem.

Subsequent readings showed me that focusing on raising one's vibration would not only lead to physical, emotional, and spiritual health, but could actually prevent illness. I was so excited by this revelation, I didn't realize I was becoming a true healer.

As word of my readings spread, I became known as a Medical Intuitive healer because I worked on the mind-body-spirit connection and helped raise a person's vibration.

So when Alicia came to my office and said she couldn't get pregnant, I wanted to know why. I didn't need to know about her test results or failed in vitro fertilizations or how her doctors said she would never get pregnant and should adopt. I needed to know what her chakras looked like. I needed to know if tribal beliefs, toxic thoughts, or other people's energy were cluttering up her energy field. I needed to identify the emotional patterns that were lowering her vibration so her womb could not support new life.

My reading was short and sweet. I saw nothing terribly remarkable in Alicia's energy field, just a few minor indications of childhood traumas. Her field had good color — soft pinks, greens, and lavenders — but its edges, instead of being smooth, looked jagged and spiky.

Physically, Alicia was healthy as a horse. She didn't need to adopt a child: There was nothing wrong with her reproductive system. Emotionally, though, I picked up several patterns: unwillingness to express anger, the need for control (which she tried to get by telling her husband what to do), and the fear of what might happen if things were not perfect. She had a "polite indifference," as she put it, to God. She had stopped praying because her prayers for a child had not been answered. She felt that God was ignoring her.

In regard to her current situation, Alicia was struggling with feelings of helplessness, repressed anger, and hostility. She also felt very alone in her marriage. Her husband had a fear of intimacy. The more distant he was, the more hurt and angry she became. When I read Alicia's energy system, I saw that part of the reason she could not get pregnant was that she felt completely disconnected from her husband. Her soul knew it would be unhealthy for a child to be born into a situation like this.

Alicia's emotional issues were centered in her second chakra. This energy center is just above the pubic bone, and it is

Thoughts and Feelings That Raise Your Vibration...

◆ Expect the best.
◆ Love someone.
◆ Laugh.
◆ Don't hold grudges.
◆ Be generous.
◆ Accept people as they are.
◆ Act with kindness.

...or Lower It

◆ Be cynical.
◆ Resent someone.
◆ Complain.
◆ Get mad and stay mad.
◆ Be selfish.
◆ Be intolerant and prejudiced.
◆ Be rude to someone.

about one's most significant relationship. When a person doesn't feel inherently worthwhile or lovable, she tries to make her significant other love her by manipulating him. She might not realize it's manipulation. But if she sacrifices her own needs, hides her anger, denies that anything is wrong – or does anything to win or keep the love she thinks she doesn't deserve – it's manipulation.

This is the only way some people feel loved, worthwhile, powerful, and in control. This is what Alicia was doing with her husband. Ironically – and sadly – manipulating others only gets you approval, not love. It also drains energy from your second chakra. If all of Alicia's second-chakra energy was being used to manipulate her husband into loving her, what was left to support a fertile environment for a new life? Nothing.

By the time Alicia came to see me, she was depressed, angry, and desperate. She would have done anything I told her, including swinging a plastic chicken over her head while chanting and inhaling incense, if it would have helped her to become pregnant. So when I discussed a plan that would lead to conception she was eager to comply without hesitation or complaint. First, I told her that she should stop trying to get pregnant for three months. Making love was fine, but not with the goal of conceiving. Then I outlined some specific things she and her husband could do. Alicia and I used a number of energetic and spiritual techniques to heal her emotional pattern of being a victim: someone who is wounded and retreats into unspoken anger, helplessness, fear, and the need to control. Alicia's husband worked on learning how to be present and intimate with her.

Eventually they both took responsibility for the emotional patterns they had been living, changed them, and – before the three months were up – had the joy of discovering that Alicia was pregnant.

Before scientists found biochemical evidence of the mind-body connection, people used to laugh (or sneer) at the idea that an aspect of a person's physical health, such as her ability to conceive or her resistance to disease, could be affected by her thoughts or feelings. Now we know better. Key to this discovery was the work of Dr. Candace Pert, a neuroscientist and former chief of brain chemistry at the National Institute of Mental Health. Dr. Pert identified the chemicals in our bodies whose job is to communicate what we are feeling emotionally to our cells.

These "molecules of emotion," as Pert calls them, are amino acid chains called neuropeptides. They carry their messages (such as contentment, sadness, or embarrassment) to *all* our cells, including those of our bones, muscles, and internal organs. In fact, neuropeptides literally put our minds – that is, our thoughts, emotions, and beliefs – into every cell in our bodies. They are the hyphen in "the mind-body connection."

What happens when these emotional messages reach our cells? Our cells respond. For example, researchers at the University of Wisconsin who were studying patterns of brain activity have shown that positive states of mind like happiness and surprise enhance the immune system, while those of negative emotions like anger, sadness, and fear weaken it.

These findings confirm my experience in the E.R. Consider Dora and her appendicitis, for example. If you ask anyone who has had appendicitis, she will probably tell you she was carrying tremendous stress and felt threatened by something or someone just before her attack.

Dora's emotional state – fear for her life – explains what I saw in her chakra system. As you'll recall, her root chakra looked like it had a black hole. This is the sign that a chakra is shut down. A healthy, open chakra looks light, not dark. It feels alive and energetic. When I put my hand over the chakra, I can feel its energy moving. When one of your energy centers shuts down, there is less life force flowing to the surrounding organs, which leaves them open to disease. Thus your chakras get "sick" before your physical body does.

The overall energy of your body (this includes your thoughts, feelings, beliefs, and attitudes) produces a vibration that can be read in your chakras and your energy field. The emotions attached to your thoughts significantly contribute to your overall vibration or chakra health.

Positive thoughts and feelings raise the frequency of your vibration, as do good feelings like high self-esteem, love, trust, generosity, and happiness. Negative thoughts and feelings like anger, pessimism, hopelessness, the need for validation, narrow-mindedness, and cynicism lower the frequency at which your energy vibrates.

Fear is the most harmful emotion of all. It not only lowers your vibration, it weakens your immune system because it triggers a fight-or-flight response every time you feel it, sending a surge of adrenaline into your bloodstream. The adrenaline speeds up your heartbeat, constricts your blood vessels, and increases your blood pressure, all of which gear you up for your fight or flight. But when we force our immune system to constantly gear up like this, it wears down and loses its ability to respond in a healthy way when we really do need it. So every time a person says, "Heart disease runs in my family," and feels the fear inherent in that statement, he is actually *creating* his own predisposition to heart disease: His statements are triggering a repeated, though subtle, fight-or-flight response, which eventually will undermine his immune system.

In addition, conflicting thoughts and feelings drain you because you are in an energetic tug of war that divides you; supporting two opposing causes is exhausting. This too lowers your overall vibration. For example, if you believe you are lovable, but deep down aren't sure if you really deserve to be loved, this constant conflict will deplete your energy and shut down your chakra system. Many times people who appear to have it all are actually trapped in conflicting beliefs and emotions. They may not realize it, though, because it's happening on an unconscious level.

When I scan someone's energy field, I also see his predominant belief about himself. This is crucial information because your attitudes and beliefs also play a role in raising or lowering your vibration. An event can be perceived as positive or negative based upon the spin you put on it. Your attitudes and beliefs determine that spin. If you believe you are a failure, being passed over for promotion to supervisor will reinforce that belief and contribute to an overall negative attitude about life, such as "There's no point in trying." If you believe you are a valuable employee, being passed over for promotion to supervisor will simply make you wonder whether that position would have really been a good match (maybe you are more of an independent thinker than a team leader) or whether you are working for the wrong company.

In the first instance, your low-vibration belief about yourself (*I am a failure*) has cemented itself into a low-vibration attitude about life (*There's no point in trying*), which is the classic self-fulfilling belief. It's also a belief that can be very dangerous to your health because it could prevent you from even trying to get well. In the second case, your high-vibration belief (*I am very good at what I do*) has been reflected in one of two high-vibration attitudes (*That was not the best job for me after all*, or *I deserve to work for a better company, one that recognizes my abilities*). You could say that this belief, too, is a self-fulfilling prophecy, because it would spur you to take positive action.

Never, never underestimate the power of your beliefs and attitudes. In his work at Stanford, Dr. Bruce Lipton has found that the nature of your beliefs about yourself and your attitudes about the world can affect — even alter — the genetic makeup of your cells. You can't get more powerful than that.

What this discovery means is that science now supports what good Medical Intuitives have always said: Your genes *do not* irreversibly determine who you are — or what diseases you will get.

Now You Know...

◆ Your thoughts, feelings, attitudes, and beliefs have a powerful effect on your energy system, and therefore on your physical health. PAGE 52.

◆ Positive thoughts and feelings raise your vibration. Negative ones lower it and "invite" illness into your energy system and then into your body. PAGE 53.

◆ Raising your vibration leads to physical, emotional and spiritual health, and can help you conceive. PAGE 54.

◆ You have a choice about whether to have negative or positive thoughts and feelings. You have a choice about whether to put a negative or positive spin on the events in your adult life. PAGE 54.

◆ The choices you make can affect every cell in your body, even at the genetic level. PAGE 55.

◆ Your genes do not irreversibly determine your health or illness. PAGE 55.

CHAPTER 7

Caution: Positive Thinking Can Be Harmful to Your Health

Even in the world of energy, thinking something
doesn't make it so. You have to believe it, too.

Positive thoughts can cause illness.

Does this statement makes you uncomfortable? It should, because it's true.

How can this be so? For years, practitioners of complementary medicine have been recommending we combat illness by reciting positive affirmations. What's more, I just told you that both science and my own medical intuition testify to the fact that your thoughts and feelings impact your health. So how can your *positive* thoughts possibly cause illness?

Because you don't really believe them.

Perhaps you've done the exercise where you stand in front of the mirror and say, "I love you." Or the one where you look into your own eyes and say three things you like about yourself. Or you make it a practice to program your day by beginning it with the words, "It's going to be a great day!"

Next time you do one of these things, ask yourself this: Do you *mean* it?

If so, your positive affirmations are indeed a good thing. I have clients who came in with illnesses who look in the mirror many times a day and affirm they are getting healthy. Through their work with me, they have changed the energy behind their words. They believe them. This has resulted in chemotherapy patients raising their white blood cell counts, seeing their tumors shrink, and having their blood tests return to normal. When they mean it, it works.

How can I tell if someone truly means the positive words they are saying? I watch the energy of her words start at her crown chakra, travel down her chakra system to the root chakra, then run back up again to her crown. If I see the energy of her words stop in a particular chakra, I know there is an emotional issue keeping those words from being true for that client – no matter how many times she repeats them. Once I've identified the blocked chakra, I know immediately what the problem is, often to the consternation and disbelief of the client.

Take John, for example. At thirty-four, John wanted nothing more than a loving relationship leading to marriage. At least, that's what he'd been telling himself for the past ten years. One look at John's third chakra (the center of self-esteem, confidence, and courage) told me all I needed to know. It was completely blocked. John had no self-esteem. His predominant belief was that he wasn't worth loving.

When I told John what I saw, it was hard for him to hear because he had been affirming for years that he deserved a loving relationship. I explained that the words of his affirmation were like a whisper on a lake at twilight: nearly imperceptible. To translate that in terms of energy: John's cells couldn't "hear" him when he affirmed his desire for a relationship – the energy behind his words was too low to register. Energetically, what they "heard" instead was his deep-down belief that he wasn't worthy of love.

At first, John didn't think this was really the reason that he hadn't found the woman of his dreams. It was too simple. So I asked him to say out loud the words "I am not lovable." He did – and was shocked at how strongly he could feel those words resonating through his body. I could see the energy of his statement run down and back up his chakra system like lightning. Then I asked him to say out loud his usual affirmation, "I deserve a good relationship." When he did so, John was suddenly aware of the elusive and hollow ring of his words when the energy behind them died as it reached his third chakra.

Having this experience was John's first step in learning to feel the energy behind his own words. It required profound honesty on his part. Fortunately, he was more interested in having a loving relationship than proving me wrong. To this day I teach people how to discern when what they say they want is in alignment – or in conflict – with their energy. When they learn how to identify what kind of energy is behind their affirmations (in John's case it was low self-esteem), they can heal their blocks and make their affirmations come true. John did. He's now happily married!

The same principle holds true for people who are ill and say they want to get better. If their words get stuck in a particular chakra, the energy behind those words just drains away, and I can see their ambivalence to getting well. This ambivalence can be caused by trauma, low self-worth, feeling trapped and resigned to their illness, or feeling it's easier to die than to stay here and deal with life's problems.

Awareness of one's true feelings is the first step in the three-step healing process I guide my clients through.

1. **Awareness** – Becoming aware that some of the positive things you believe about yourself are not true, and understanding what your unconscious beliefs and motivations really are. It is vital when you are doing this work not to become judgmental or critical of yourself, but to simply notice, from a neutral perspective, where you are investing your energy. It is either bringing you the results you want or the results you don't want. The more you beat yourself up for what you are learning about yourself, the slower your healing will be!

2. **Ownership** – Claiming ownership of the dysfunctional ways in which your deepest beliefs about yourself are manifesting themselves in your daily life. What daily choices do you make that are driven by your buried beliefs? Again, resist the urge to say, "I can't believe I do that! How stupid!" or "What's wrong with me?" Castigating or punishing yourself for what you see will just slow you down.

3. **Action** – Taking action to heal the unconscious, life-draining belief that is blocking you from living a free, healthy, and happy life by either rewriting or letting go of the belief.

This three-part process is the essence of healing. It's crucial to identify the unconscious beliefs that are getting in your way. They are carried in your energy field, where they lower your vibration. A low vibration opens a direct line to illness, emotional difficulty, and all sorts of misfortune. Better, like John, to own those beliefs and heal them than sign up for a lifetime of frustration because you don't want to believe they're really there.

So how about you? How much of your energy is in alignment with your words? When you look in the mirror and say, "I love all of me *unconditionally*," is it true? You probably want to say yes. But before you bet the ranch on it, listen to some of the common behaviors that show the difference between loving oneself and loving oneself *unconditionally*.

◆   ◆   ◆

Barbara used to feel sick as a dog for several days after chemotherapy, yet she still got up early every morning to make breakfast for her husband. She fought back nausea, dizziness, and extreme fatigue, but when her husband asked her how she was feeling, Barbara smiled and replied, "Pretty good." The truth was, making her husband breakfast wiped her out. She had to stay in bed for most of the rest of the day, fighting to get her chemotherapy-induced nausea under control.

If Barbara's husband called from work to ask if they needed anything from the store, she would tell him, "Just a carton of milk," even though the household needed groceries. The sad irony was that having a variety of food in the house was especially important for Barbara. The taste buds of people who are having chemotherapy get altered by the drugs, and they can only eat certain things at certain times of the day. And it's crucial that they eat so they can keep their weight up.

But because Barbara didn't want to put her husband out, she would only ask him to pick up milk and would do without the only foods she could stand to eat. Barbara felt that because her husband worked hard all day and took care of her, she shouldn't burden him anymore.

The reality was, Barbara, who claimed to like herself well enough, didn't think she was worth much and wouldn't have dreamed of asking for what she needed if she thought it would inconvenience someone. By being "nice" and not asking for too much, she thought she was more lovable. Specifically, she thought she could make him keep loving her even though deep down she knew she wasn't worth loving.

Now, people who think they are not lovable don't generally walk around saying so. But that subconscious belief is present in their energy system. It drives their choices, lowers their vibration, and affects them every day. Most people are not aware of these beliefs, especially if they have accomplished a lot in the world. How could you think you are unworthy of love, after all, when you have a degree, a great job, and think you have a great relationship, or you're famous, you support the community, take care of yourself, maybe even speak up when you need things?

Dig a little deeper. Look at your unconscious behavior, and ask yourself what is motivating it. For example, notice how you reply when someone offers you something. When you go out to lunch with a friend and she wants to buy you lunch, do you have a hard time accepting her generosity? Do you fight over the check? Do you only give in by saying, "Okay, but next time it's my turn to pay"?

An underlying sense of worthlessness makes it difficult for you to graciously receive. How do you react when someone gives you an expensive gift? Do you feel uncomfortable? Do you say, "Oh, it's wonderful—thank you!" or do you protest, "Oh, you shouldn't have" or even "It's wonderful, but I can't possibly accept it"?

Keep an eye on your actions and listen to your replies when people are kind to you. Notice how you respond. These responses may be automatic, made without thought, but they reveal your belief that you're not worth it – even if you started the day by looking in the mirror and saying, "I love you." What's more, your true feelings of worthlessness are being carried to every cell in your body by neuropeptides, those little chemical messengers I talked about in the previous chapter.

Remember that I asked you to *notice* your actions and responses, not judge them. Becoming aware of your beliefs and actions does not mean bashing yourself. That only makes you feel worse!

I often remind my clients that energy is neutral. This means that there is no point in feeling ashamed or guilty because you have thoughts and feelings that have lowered your vibration. Having a low vibration isn't morally bad; having a high vibration isn't morally good. "Low" and "high" simply describe the frequencies of these vibrations, not one's moral worth. So notice whether your automatic reactions are evidence that you feel worthless. If they are, make the choice to change. It's crucial that you do.

If you continue feeling worthless, these feelings will block your growth and open your body to disease. Negative feelings about yourself lower your vibration and resonate with illness, whether that illness be simple aches and pains, a persistent feeling of exhaustion, or a more serious condition like cancer. Without reading your energy, I can't tell you what physical problems you will suffer, but I can guarantee you that having even a slight sense of worthlessness will have negative repercussions on your health.

I am going to tell you how to create a sense of true self-worth, but before I do, I want to offer an option to those of you who are reluctant to change your thinking to believe you are truly lovable. Sometimes it can be a hard choice. Maybe you still carry the energy of a wounded child. Your parents may have taught you not to blow your own horn. Pride could be preventing you from admitting you need to change your behavior. Or you might be getting some benefit from feeling worthless. For example, your friends may have learned to constantly reassure or encourage you, and their attention feels good.

If any of these are true for you, I recommend giving yourself permission to be conflicted. By owning the awareness that part of you wants to be lovable and part you isn't sure you deserve it, you stop the internal tug of war that is draining your energy. Instead of fighting it, repeatedly say aloud: "I fully love and accept all of me, even though I don't believe I am lovable." You will feel your internal tension literally melt away because you are accepting the part of you that doesn't feel deserving.

When that statement becomes easy to say, it's time to begin your affirmations anew. By this I mean, say those affirmations even if you don't believe them right now. The key is to *keep an open mind* about whether they are true or not. Stay neutral on the subject. See what you discover. You'll be able to feel the difference in your body when you say "I love myself" with a neutral attitude vs. saying "I love myself" when inside you think you're useless. The first gives you room to grow, to discover what happens when you "act as if." (It can be surprisingly effective.) In addition, taking a genuine wait-and-see approach to feeling lovable will not lower your vibration and make you prone to illness. Lying to yourself about it will.

Why do most people feel worthless? What's underneath it? Why does Barbara cook her husband breakfast when she feels so sick? Why does someone have a hard time receiving but take great pleasure in giving?

What about you? Do you think of others before you think of yourself? Do you silence your own needs, yet take care of another's? Why?

Part of the reason may be that you were raised this way. If so, your parents were just passing on their own sense of worthlessness to you.* The real cause is that you are afraid. You are scared senseless that if you don't take care of other people, they won't like you or love you, and they will leave you.

Let the truth of this idea sink in. Don't fight it by becoming defensive. I can hear you saying, "I know my husband loves me and wouldn't leave me." Or, "I know I could say anything to my friends, and they would still like me." I agree that you know this on an intellectual level. But the key is, do you really believe it? Do you feel the energy of your words run through your chakra system? Deep in your heart, the answer might be no. Or, deep in your heart, you aren't sure – and you are scared to find out the truth.

Too many people were not loved unconditionally as children. They were loved for what they did, not who they were. This sets them up for a life of doing, doing, doing in the vain hope of earning another's love. Why do I say their hopes are in vain? Because the best you can earn by *doing* things for others is approval, a sense of obligation, or gratitude. (The first two you don't want, and the third won't do you any good unless you have the ability to receive it.) The truth is, you can't *earn* unconditional love, but you can give it to yourself.

Dig deep, my friend, and see what lurks in your subconscious mind. All those fears and worries about whether others really love you can strangle you. They can keep you from loving yourself unconditionally. They can also keep you from loving someone else: When you feel unworthy of love, you distance yourself from others; you are lonely, disconnected – and alone.

What are some of these positive thoughts that can cause illness? For Barbara, it's thinking that she feels up to cooking

---

* It's important to distinguish between being taught to care for others and being taught to care for others *at the expense of our own well-being*. It's the second one that leads to feelings of worthlessness.

breakfast, going grocery shopping, or staying up to talk when all she wants to do is sleep. It's acting really positive when deep down she is angry and scared that she is so sick. It's faking it. It's creating a façade that says, "I'm feeling well enough to do this for my family." It's abandoning yourself for another under the guise of, "I love you and want to do this for you." It's going to lunch and thinking how nice it feels to take your turn buying your friend lunch – when underneath you are simply scared that she might not see you as an equal if you don't reciprocate her generous gesture.

Worst of all, this kind of "positive" thinking – the façade you present to the world – prevents you from feeling your true feelings. When you don't feel your fear or anger, it doesn't just dissipate. It builds up inside. It lowers your vibration because you have to devote energy to keeping it buried. And the farther down you stuff those feelings, the more potential there is to resonate with illness. Why are so many people afflicted with fatigue, boredom, and chronic aches and pains? Because their true feelings are sapping all their energy, while they smile and make merry for the world.

Here are some more examples of "positive" behavior that can be harmful to your health. See if you recognize yourself in any of them.

- ◆ Have you ever been sick and had someone ask how you were? Did you tell the truth? Or did you respond with "Fine," "Feeling better, thanks," or "Not bad," even though you felt terrible?

- ◆ Are you honest about what you feel with some friends, but not others because you are afraid of them judging you?

- ◆ Do you keep your troubles to yourself because you

don't want to burden your friends or family?

♦ Are you known as a great listener?

♦ Do you make sure everyone else is content before seeing to your own needs?

♦ Do you attend social engagements when you'd rather stay home?

♦ Do you work overtime even if you are exhausted, because your co-workers need help?

♦ Do you get angry sometimes because people don't seem to consider your feelings and needs?

♦ Do you feel taken advantage of?

♦ Are you a habitual caretaker?

♦ Do you keep your true feelings to yourself?

If you answered yes or sometimes to *any* of these questions, it's time to dig deep and let your feelings out. While it may seem frightening at first, think of the benefits. Ask yourself, "Can I afford *not* to feel my true feelings? Can I afford to drain my energy by keeping up such pretenses? Am I ready and willing to make choices that will enhance – and extend – my life?"

It's up to you. You can continue to act nice and please others at your own expense, or you can vow to act in your own best interests by telling the truth about how you feel. When you do, your sense of self-worth will skyrocket. You won't be in danger of having positive thoughts that can make you ill. *Your* positive thoughts will be genuine.

Now You Know...

◆ Positive thoughts about yourself will not raise your vibration if, in your heart of hearts, you don't really believe them. PAGE 57.

◆ Many people secretly harbor feelings of worthlessness that dramatically lower their vibration. PAGE 62.

◆ They hide their supposed worthlessness by acting nice and doing things for others. PAGE 61.

◆ Feeling worthless is guaranteed to have negative repercussions on your health. PAGE 63.

◆ Healing is a three-step process consisting of awareness, ownership, and action. First you must become aware of the unconscious beliefs that lower your vibration. Then you take ownership of the ways in which these beliefs are interfering with your life. Finally you take action to change them. PAGE 60.

◆ Speaking the truth about your needs and your feelings will enhance and extend your life because it raises your vibration by dramatically increasing your sense of self-worth. PAGE 63.

CHAPTER 8

Healing the Beliefs
That Drain Your Energy

If an organism "perceives" a stress that is not actually there,
that misperception can...change the genes
to accommodate the "belief."
— *Cellular Biologist Bruce Lipton, Ph.D.*

When I read your energy field, I can see your predominant negative belief about yourself, how you came to develop that belief, and how it has sabotaged your hopes and dreams. I can also see exactly what you need to do to change that belief and what your life will look like when you do.

Your predominant negative belief is found in your energy field, and it influences almost everything you say and do. It is a reflection of how you feel about your personal worth. Some examples of predominant negative beliefs include *I am not pretty, I am not lovable, I'm stupid,* or *I'm a failure.* Interestingly, some of

69

the most successful people I've met carry the belief *I'm a failure,* and some of the most well-liked individuals carry *I'm not lovable.* These beliefs drive them to achieve beyond all expectations, yet they still feel that they never do enough. They have to give endlessly for fear that if they stop giving, people won't love them anymore.

These beliefs are generally not spoken aloud or even consciously known, yet to me they shout from your energy field. When I report the predominant belief, some people sigh with relief because their terrible secret is finally out in the open, while others defiantly say it isn't so – but soon admit the truth.

How did you come to develop your predominant negative belief? Sometimes it can be as simple as a passing statement from someone in authority, such as a teacher who says, "You'll never amount to anything." Or an older sibling who says, "You're ugly." Sometimes these negative beliefs result from traumatic events such as verbal, emotional, or sexual abuse, the loss of a parent, or being married to someone who repeatedly degrades and denigrates you.

Beliefs like this can sabotage your hopes and dreams. If you believe that you are not pretty, smart, or lovable, your self-esteem will suffer. Having no sense of self-value will inhibit you from exploring new relationships or careers. A pattern will ensue whereby you give up your heart's desire because you believe your goal is not attainable. Even if you do reach some of your goals, you never feel complete or content. Instead you are restless and somewhat anxious. These states slowly and steadily drain your energy, resulting in a lower vibration.

Many of my clients come to me after long years of psychotherapy where they're used to exploring and examining exactly where all their limiting beliefs came from. While I can see the events that precipitated your negative belief, it is more important to heal them than explore them. The bottom line is, these beliefs are draining you and inhibiting you from leading a full and happy life. My goal is to show you how to change them *quickly*. This shocks people who believe that it takes years of work to change how they feel about themselves.

A second type of belief that can drain your energy is called a **tribal belief.** This kind of belief is adopted from your family, teachers, and religious institutions because

Tribal Belief

An unconscious assumption instilled during childhood by your family, teachers, or religious training, such as *Girls aren't as smart as boys* or *Men owe it to their families to work hard and earn a lot of money.*

Most tribal beliefs are energy-draining. Also, they don't *feel* like beliefs; to you, they are inescapable facts. Tribal beliefs reside in the root chakra, where they chip away at your sense of safety in the world and your desire to live.

the people in these groups make up your "tribe." The purpose of the tribe is to protect you, educate you, and raise you to adulthood so that you can become a useful member of it. The purpose of tribal beliefs is to bind the group together through a common belief system. Unfortunately, many of these beliefs are misguided or just plain erroneous. The biggest problem with tribal beliefs, however, is that you may not even realize they are *beliefs*. You may think they are facts.

Here are some examples of the tribal beliefs that people I have worked with have had:

- ◆ A woman can never be as successful or as powerful as a man.

- ◆ Money equals power.

- ◆ Don't let anyone get the better of you.

◆ You can't be happy unless your family is happy.

◆ Father (or Mother) knows best.

◆ If your mother gives you up for adoption, it's because you are damaged goods.

◆ Secrets should stay in the family.

◆ Don't take risks.

◆ You are a born sinner.

◆ If your mother doesn't love you, no one will.

◆ Suffering is noble.

◆ Always take care of others before yourself.

◆ Stay small and you'll stay safe.

Tribal beliefs like these affect your health because they put you into a conflict between following tribal law or listening to your soul. This conflict drains your energy, thus lowering your vibration. For example, most people realize that worrying is both anxiety-producing and a waste of time. Yet, if tribal law says that you should worry or that love is expressed through worrying, you face a conflict. You can follow tribal law and be worried and wrung out, or you can give up worrying because you know it's a waste of time. Why is there a conflict in giving up worrying? Just try visiting your tribe, which is busy worrying, while you are feeling peaceful. They will think you don't care.

Or imagine your tribe says you should get married and have children, but your soul yearns for an exciting career. Regardless of how exciting a career you pursue, you will always feel "less than" around your family because your sister has children but you don't. What about the conflict you would feel if your soul knew that your marriage was over and dead, but the tribal belief was that marriage is forever, no matter what!

When you reject the tribal way and choose to follow your soul, survival issues arise. You feel less and less safe within the tribal unit. The conflict you feel blocks energy from entering your all-important root chakra. While this energy center is located near your genitals (where the inseams of your pants meet, to be exact), it does not govern sexuality. It is linked to issues much more basic to your survival than your sexuality. Your sense of safety in the world, your desire to be alive, and your level of comfort with your role (or absence of a role) in your family affects the health of your root chakra. Most important of all, your root chakra is the depository for your tribal beliefs.

Tribal beliefs are almost always unconscious until you make a deliberate effort to uncover them. Depending on the nature of your tribe, these beliefs can be positive and beneficial or negative and harmful. The latter restrict your life force and lower your self-esteem, which lowers your vibration and opens up your energy system to illness, conflict, struggle, depression, or unhappiness.

When you read that list of tribal beliefs I made, did you think how ridiculous or old-fashioned they were? Did you wonder how anyone could possibly think that way? Remember, these beliefs are not the products of your rational mind. They are unconscious. You do not know they exist. In fact, you often *think* that you believe just the opposite. In my work I am constantly amazed at the discrepancy between what most people think they believe and what they really believe.

The power of a toxic tribal belief to shape and control your life is nothing short of shocking. The good news is, the reverse is also true. I have seen people's entire lives start to make sense to them once they uncover their tribal beliefs. A man in one of my workshops who was suffering from cardiac problems secondary to diabetes told the group that "a good man never quits working, even if he is very, very sick." Taken to its logical extreme, this means that a good man does not stop working until he is dead.

Since Bill wanted to be a good man who provided for his wife and four children, he could not cut back his work either at his job or around the house, no matter how much his body needed a rest. He left the workshop unable to break free from the hold of this vicious belief. I went home feeling sad that such a wonderful human being had decided to literally work himself to death.

But Bill came back for a couple of individual sessions, during which we talked about his attachment to this toxic tribal belief. I told him it was time to choose between living or dying. When I saw Bill a few months later, I hardly recognized him. He had begun an exercise program, lost forty pounds, was working less so he could take time for himself, and had decided to take early retirement. He looked like a new man – and in fact, he was.

These changes came easily and naturally once Bill let go and changed his old tribal belief. Even his father, who had inadvertently taught Bill to think this way, was thrilled with the changes in his son. Even more exciting, Bill's own son, a boy of thirteen, is now being taught a decidedly different way of defining himself as a man. He will not inherit the tribal belief that nearly killed his father.

At the start of this chapter, I said that energy-draining beliefs can be taught to you by the "tribe" or they can be the result of a traumatic experience. Whether one's toxic beliefs are tribal or traumatic in origin, they set in motion long-term, unhealthy patterns of behavior.

The things about yourself that you don't own (usually because you are not aware of them) constitute your shadow. We all have one. Your shadow is the buried and unconscious part of yourself that is running the show. It's what drives your behavior. It is the part that you have disavowed or disowned.

Uncovering what's in your shadow is crucial to your physical, emotional, and spiritual health because your shadow can prevent you from healing. No matter what efforts you make to change your lifestyle or your beliefs, your true motives – which lie hidden in your shadow – will still be driving your behavior and will eventually sabotage all your good work. I have seen this again and again in my practice. Unless one hundred percent of you is committed to changing your beliefs and healing, you won't get well and stay well. It's like trying to clear your garden of weeds by chopping them off at ground level. Pretty soon, the undamaged roots send up new shoots and strangle all your flowers.

Toxic beliefs hate the light of day. They thrive in the shadow Once you have exposed them by becoming conscious of them, you can choose whether to change them or not. Sad to say, not everyone truly wants to heal. It's a dilemma I often see. A client will say, "I don't want to be sick and in pain," but if a deeper part of him feels as though he deserves to be sick and in pain, or if he insists on holding on to a tribal belief that says suffering is noble, guess who wins? A person's shadow always overrides any healer.

Jack is sixty-one and a perpetual student. He loves to read and discuss ideas and philosophies, especially about God. When Jack came to consult me, he appeared easygoing and affable. But when I scanned his energy system, I saw he was being followed by a shadow of himself, a doppelganger. His energy field was hazy and gray, which is indicative of someone who is thinking about dying, is getting ready to die, or is thoroughly depressed. In scanning his physical body, I saw prostate cancer, but it wasn't so far along that it couldn't be cured.

"Jack," I began, "have you had a checkup lately?"

He looked at me and smiled. "I know I have cancer."

I was struck by how unconcerned he seemed about his diagnosis. When I scanned his emotional body, I saw that Jack felt trapped and resigned. He was eagerly anticipating that death would release him from his unhappy life.

"Jack, if your life stayed the same, would you want to live?"

He thought for a moment. "No, I'm ready to go."

"Your prostate cancer isn't that bad. You don't have metastasis. It's beatable."

"I guess that's good news," he replied unemotionally.

"I'll tell you what," I said. "I'll tell you what your life looks like, identify the patterns that make you feel like dying, and show you some choices you can make to change it all. Okay?"

He accepted my challenge.

"First," I began, "you are sooooo pissed off! You hold in your anger, never speak up for your needs, and are filled with resentment toward your wife and children. Plus you hate confrontation. How am I doing?"

Jack merely smiled, so I continued.

"You feel powerless, resigned, and trapped. You believe that dying is the easy way out."

He nodded.

"Your fear of being alone has prevented you from taking risks or fully living life in a passionate way."

Now Jack took a deep breath. "You're good," he said genially.

"Hold on, I'm not done yet! You like to be a peacemaker, which traps you in the middle of people's disagreements, and you are in a spiritual crisis. God is only an intellectual concept to you. You scramble around gathering information about God, but you never take the plunge and pray...."

"And you hate your father for leaving your mother."

Jack looked at me like I was from Mars. Then a smile slowly crept over his face.

"You nailed me," he laughed. "You can really see all that?"

"And more," I replied.

Jack's father, who was a meek man, had been constantly berated by Jack's mother for being "boring," meaning he was not athletic. Once while screaming at her husband, she turned to Jack and said, "I'm right, you know. Your father is a weakling." When Jack attempted to defend his father, she got in his face and said, "Don't ever disagree with me when I'm right." The unspoken consequence was more frightening than any actual threat could have been. Jack learned to avoid confrontation at all costs. He became a peacemaker. At home, he learned to be invisible and stay out of his parents' fights.

Jack's entire chakra system was blocked, producing tremendous fatigue and an overall listlessness toward life. He did not have **magnetics** for the life he was leading, but he was too scared to say anything. In fact, Jack lacked passion or excitement about anything. He lived mostly in his head and rarely dared to engage others with any feelings.

Magnetics

Magnetics is a strong resonance for a specific situation. It can neither be forced nor faked. When you have magnetics for something, you feel vibrant and alive when you do it. Your vibration is high. You are acting in alignment with your soul's wishes. You can tell when you have magnetics for a relationship or a profession because you are energized by being in it.

When you lose magnetics for something, it exhausts you to do it. Your vibration drops. You are swimming upstream, ignoring your spiritual guidance. You can tell you have lost magnetics for a relationship or a profession because you feel drained by it.

Now his tremendous fear of losing the love and approval of his wife kept him immobilized, even though his soul was shouting at him to change his life by being *real* with people. His second chakra was hemorrhaging energy because he was manipulating others to win their approval. He swallowed his needs out of fear of being rejected. This energetic impotence lowered his vibration enough to resonate with prostate cancer.

The reason for Jack's doppelganger was that he presented a façade to the world that was quite different from who he really was. To others, Jack appeared likeable, gentle, and cerebral, but inside, the real Jack was angry and resentful most of the time.

Jack's case is a sad one. He chose to continue the status quo, even though it meant dying. It was easier somehow. His conscious choice to stay in his situation overrode any help or energetic healing I could offer him. As a result, Jack died years before his time.

❖   ❖   ❖

Mary was fifty-three when she came to see me, but judging by her appearance, she could easily have been seventy-three. She looked worn out, as if she had led a difficult and trying life. Energetically she had a very low vibration. Mary told me about her fatigue and her many allergies and said she desperately wanted to be well again. She also had mood swings and felt a distinct apathy for life. Mary's older brother used to fondle her when she was nine. When she told her mother, she felt humiliated by the reply she got: "Boys will be boys." When Mary said how much she hated her brother touching her private parts, her mother told her to be quiet and offer it up to God, who loves us even more when we suffer.

So Mary learned to suffer well, suffer silently, and always give her power away to men. By age fifty-three, she had mastered the trauma of her brother's abuse and her mother's callous reaction to it by unconsciously deciding that she had brought it on herself: She believed she was a horrible person who deserved to suffer. She hadn't been in a relationship in twenty years, had no friends, and felt very unlikable.

Mary sat quietly until my scan was complete.

"On a scale of one to ten," I asked her, "how would you say you like yourself?"

"Oh, I like myself a lot," Mary responded with faint enthusiasm.

Energetic Blueprint

Your energetic blueprint contains information about your beliefs, your perceptions about yourself and others, your connection with God, and your vibration. In short, it is a map that shows where you are putting your energy and whether those places are life-enhancing or not.

"Hmmm. How about if I tell you what I see, and you simply listen. I'm not here to convince you of anything, but simply to report your **energetic blueprint** to you. Anything I say that you don't like, you can throw in the wastebasket on the way out." Mary nodded.

"First, I see that you constantly berate yourself over every little thing. You hate the fact that you aren't perfect, even though you try hard to be so. There is so much chatter in your mind, you can barely think, and most of it is self-denigrating. You give your power away to any man in your path. You push people away by being a know-it-all who tries to solve their problems. You do this to build up your self-esteem, but it doesn't work."

I took a breath and continued before she could argue.

"You love to complain about your life but take no responsibility for what it looks like. You love to suffer because you think it is noble. On some level you believe that suffering will expunge all of your wrongdoing – much of which is just your perception, not reality.

"There is absolutely nothing wrong with you physically, yet you continually go to doctors hoping they will find some ailment. You are not connected to your family, other people, or a Higher Power, and that scares the daylights out of you."

By now Mary looked quite shocked.

"Remember, I am not here to judge you, and I am not here to convince you of anything. I am simply asking you to go home, think about what I've said, then call me."

When Mary said she wanted to be well again, she was speaking the truth, but not the whole truth. She was conflicted about getting well because of her fear of moving forward. Therefore, getting her on medication or talking with her about her emotional issues would only be a temporary fix. What we really needed to do was trace the origin of her condition.

Mary came back and did some good work. Once she had unveiled her predominant belief that suffering was noble and understood where it came from, she could decide whether this belief was life enhancing or not. Making a conscious choice in the here and now always opens us to help from the divine. Mary is now learning how to reach out to people instead of repel them. She has quieted much of the self-critical chatter in her head, and she is exploring her shadow. In her case, the disowned parts of herself in her shadow include her brilliance, her sense of humor, and her compassionate nature.

A person's shadow does not contain only the negative traits they don't want to admit to. It contains any aspect they are blind to. For many people, that includes their gifts. Hard to believe? Go ahead and ask someone why she is amazing. I'll bet she can't tell you. She probably has a tribal belief that it's not okay to blow

HEALING THE BELIEFS THAT DRAIN YOUR ENERGY

her own horn.

Owning your shadow – the good, the bad, and the ugly – is a necessity if you want to heal on all levels. Each of your chakras is affected by a particular aspect of your shadow. For example, exploring tribal beliefs that lower your vibration will heal your first, or root, chakra. Facing the shadow in your second chakra means admitting that you try to manipulate people to win their love or approval. Owning your abilities or gifts lets energy and light into your third chakra where self-esteem, courage, and confidence reside.

When you explore your shadow, you may not like everything you see, but you always have the choice to change it. You can go from being a victim of your unconscious beliefs to living your life as an empowered, passionate, happy, and unique individual.

If you think that making a change of this magnitude takes a long time, you are in the grip of a tribal belief.

The reality is, you can do it overnight.

Now You Know...

◆ Negative thoughts, feelings, attitudes, and beliefs can result from the teachings of your family, teachers, or religion, or from being traumatized. PAGE 70.

◆ Tribal beliefs can lower your vibration. PAGE 72.

◆ Tribal beliefs are stored in your root chakra and can
  prevent a healthy flow of energy through your system.
  PAGE 73.

◆ Tribal beliefs that are in conflict with your soul will
  block your root chakra and make you feel unsafe. PAGE
  73.

◆ You can easily change your tribal beliefs once you have
  identified them. PAGE 75.

◆ Magnetics cannot be forced. PAGE 77.

CHAPTER 9

My Own Descent Into Illness

In the dark night of the soul,
bright flows the river of God.

— *St. John of the Cross*

L ife in the E.R. went on, and everything appeared to be going well. I was successful in my job, enjoyed it immensely, and received great satisfaction from it. I had a good pension package, a 401k, and five weeks of vacation a year. From the outside, it looked like I was in the groove. Inside, it was a whole 'nother story.

You see, God had clearly and unmistakably told me to leave my job and use my gift on a full-time basis. I clearly and unmistakably remember my response: "What? Are you crazy? I should leave all the trappings of success I have worked so hard to achieve? I should leave a profession I love? One I have built my entire life around?" I rationalized. I argued. I did not follow the guidance I was given.

Interestingly, God never wavered. I heard the same guidance over and over: *Leave your job*. So I did what any fun-loving, I-hate-my-guidance-because-I'm-too-scared-to-follow-it human being would do. I negotiated. I agreed to use my intuitive gift outside the E.R. by accepting private clients, but I would continue my nursing work. I convinced myself that I was following my guidance. It was bunk and I knew it.

What else can I do? I objected. I hadn't been told how to survive if I simply left my job. God had neglected to fill in the details – like where the money would come from to pay my rent. Unfortunately, that's not how guidance usually works. The details are *not* filled in. Even so, guidance is still guidance – and we will suffer if we don't listen to it. At the time, though, I didn't know just how huge that suffering could be.

God must have wondered just how stubborn I was going to be. I had managed to forget that guidance always leads us in the right direction for our lives. I didn't remember that our Higher Power always has our best interests at heart.

I was too scared to reason it out. All I knew was that I didn't want to leave a secure job and embark on an uncertain future. So I stuck to what I knew.

What happens when you do not listen to your guidance? It's simple: You begin to lose the magnetics for what you are doing. So even though I still loved my profession, I began to feel drained by my work. A series of small but powerful shifts occurred. First, the E.R. hired a new boss who was at worst pathological and at best a very unhappy and angry woman. Needless to say, she made our lives difficult. Next came a nursing shortage, complete with mandatory overtime. We were working back-to-back twelve-hour shifts, struggling to provide quality care despite dangerously low staffing levels.

Each day wore me out more than the last. I was no longer

exuberant about going to work, and I began to take sick days just to recharge myself. But did I listen to my guidance? Of course not! Like all E.R. nurses, I am very resilient. As conditions became tougher, I worked harder. Still my guidance was the same: *Leave your job and use your gift full-time.* And still I ignored it, though I knew I was out of alignment with my soul. I was too afraid of what would happen to me if I quit my job.

With no magnetics for my job, my energy took a nose-dive, my vibration dropped, and I got sick. One morning I had great difficulty getting out of bed and walking. It was the beginning of my dark night of the soul.

Looking back, I imagine the scene when God gave my angels the assignment to watch over me during this tough passage. It must have gone something like this:

God: *I have good news and I have bad news.*

(My angels exchange worried looks among themselves.)

God: *The bad news is that Christel is going to go through a dark night of the soul. Things will get pretty rocky for her. The good news is that she'll come through it — and be better than before!*

(My angels look at each other with relief but trepidation, knowing they have a tough job ahead of them.)

It got harder and harder to walk. My legs were turning numb, and I was unsteady on my feet. I was in joint pain all the time. I would drop things, like glasses of water. The vision in my right eye dimmed. I was overwhelmingly exhausted.

My diagnosis? Originally I was told I had lupus. It took them four years and many tests to diagnose multiple sclerosis. For those of you lucky enough to have no personal experience with MS, it is a chronic, cruelly unpredictable, and often progressive disease of the central nervous system that attacks and over time destroys tissues in the brain and spinal cord. There is no medical cure for it.

After being told I had MS, I fought it. Because I had periods of great health in between the flare ups, I thought, *I can beat this!* I worked harder and played harder than ever. I kept my body in shape and my mind in a positive attitude. I went on steroids, the standard treatment in those days. The regimen was six weeks on and six weeks off. The steroids would pump me up. I would feel euphoric, full of energy, and think, Yea! I'm healthy! – for those six weeks. Then I'd come off the steroids, and it would be a disaster. I was in and out of the hospital.

I began to get desperate and tried a couple of experimental treatments. The last one involved being injected with a full gram of a steroid that was supposed to blow out my immune system. Before the treatment began, I was told, "Either this will really help you, or you're going to bleed out into your brain." Twenty minutes later, I started to get a terrible headache, so I called a halt to the treatment and walked out. That was the last time I used Western medicine to alleviate my MS.

My bad days began to outweigh my good days. The sicker I got, the more my mental outlook decreased. I reached the point where I was taking so many sick days, I had to stop working. I went on sabbatical so I could still hang on to my beloved job. In just a few years, I had gone from being a supremely competent trauma nurse with a second-degree black belt in karate to being so ill I was unable to work, unable to exercise, and barely able to get out of bed in the morning.

I am sure you have heard of cases of MS where the symptoms are temporarily relieved by modern medicine. That didn't happen for me. I was focused on healing my body, but the real illness was in my spirit. I had ignored my guidance. I had lost the magnetics for my work, but still I didn't listen. What irony: There I was, an intelligent and highly experienced medical professional, looking for answers in all the wrong places.

Did I wake up and follow my guidance *then*? Nope. I turned to complementary medicine. I did a lot of praying and looked into many, many alternative treatments, including one where you got stung by about a hundred bees. (I gave that one a miss.) After a lot of string-pulling and synchronicity, I got an appointment with a well-known Medical Intuitive. He came into the room where I was waiting, took one look at me, and said without emotion, "You're going to be dead in two years." Then he walked out. It was rough, but it got my full attention. It was exactly what I needed. In that moment something inside of me snapped, and for the first time I realized that I couldn't outrun the MS.

I went home and started to put my life in order in preparation for my death. I was so fed up, so sick, and so tired of fighting, it was almost a relief. I wrote a will. I gave everything away, my art collection and all my personal possessions. I said what I needed to say to the people in my life, then I sat down to wait for death.

All right God, I thought, *I'm dying. I don't care what you do anymore. If I die or if I live, I don't care.* I had begun to surrender.

It was my first opportunity to be molded.

CHAPTER 10

Listening to God... Finally

There have been times when I think we do not desire heaven;
but more often I find myself wondering whether, in our heart
of hearts, we have ever desired anything else.

— C. S. Lewis

O ne of the ways God molds us is through synchronicity. You may not be familiar with this term, but I guarantee you are familiar with the phenomenon.

You are thinking of a friend you haven't talked to in six months, and the phone rings. It's him.

You are trying to decide whether to accept a job offer and you turn on the radio. You hear the song "Take This Job and Shove It."

You are drawn to attend a workshop on spiritual growth, even though you don't have the time. There you meet someone who can tell you where to find the one missing piece in the product line you are creating for your new business.

Synchronicity is when God puts the right door in front of you, and you just have to fall through it. In other words, it's when you have a spiritual need, and the world seems to cooperate in helping you fill it. It's also how a hardcore New York skeptic ended up in Peru with a group of New Age people searching for answers to life's mysteries.

I had never been drawn to Peru. I had no desire to go there. All I wanted to do was prepare for death. For some time now, I had been a little estranged from one of my brothers, and I didn't want to leave life with this on my conscience. My older brother – of Ouija board fame – lived in California, so I gathered my failing strength and took a plane across country to say goodbye.

One day during my visit, he looked over at me, cocked his head, and suddenly said, "I've always wanted to see Peru. Do you want to come?" All I wanted to do was bond with my brother again before I died. I didn't care where I did it. My energy level was good – my MS was in one of its inexplicable but temporary remissions – so I said yes.

We didn't want to go by ourselves, and the only tour we could get on right away was with a spiritual group. I wasn't crazy about the idea – I was still very much the empiricist and New York skeptic – but I wanted to be with my brother. Before departing, we met for a group meditation so we could meet our spirit guides. I had never heard of spirit guides, and I'm still not clear about who or what they are. My own explanation is that a spirit guide is a guardian angel who appears in the form of someone (or something) familiar and comfortable to us.

After the meditation, we shared our visions, and the spirit guides were spectacular, garnering "oohs and aaahs" from the group. Among the impressive guides people said they had met were Chief Running Bull, Gandhi, Jonas Salk, and Swami Uganami (or something like that...). Then it was my turn. In that moment, I prayed that the earth would open up, swallow me, and immediately close back up, leaving no trace of my existence. Fortunately, God has a sense of humor and ignored my silly prayer. The earth did not open up — but I was about to learn a lesson in being opened.

In those days, I was not open to things that fell under the category of "umy goomey." This is a New York term for airy fairy, New Age, woo-woo, weird, and way out there. Spirit guides came under that heading. Unimpressive spirit guides came under another heading: ridiculous.

As all eyes were upon me, waiting expectantly for the unveiling of my guide, I could only laugh. "It's a llama," I told the group.

"Oh, like the Dali Lama?" one woman said hopefully.

"No. Like a Peruvian llama. With long eyelashes."

No one stirred or blinked. They simply stared at me.

"The llama's name," I continued, "is Paco."

Slowly and silently, they nodded heads. There were no "oohs" or "aaahs" until I grabbed a piece of paper and sketched an image I had seen during the meditation. There was a triangle and within it was something that was shaped like an earthenware pot. Now they were interested. Maybe something profound had occurred, and we had all missed it. But no one recognized the image I had drawn, and they tried to hide their looks of disappointment.

This would have been a great time to quote one of my favorite authors, C. S. Lewis, who said, "We generally don't recognize when something profound is happening in our lives." But in that moment, I was the living truth of Lewis's words: All I recognized was that my prayer for the earth to mercifully open up and swallow me had not been granted. Instead we asked our spirit guides to guide us on our journey in Peru and help reveal any knowledge necessary to that journey. I prayed for any an-swers about my physical healing, but I heard nothing.

A day or so later, we were in Machu Picchu standing before a large flat rock. We were told to take turns and put our third eye (the center of the forehead) against the rock and ask a ques-tion. An answer would be forthcoming. I was the last person to try it, and I didn't follow the directions. Instead I fervently prayed for God to give me a sign that I really was supposed to quit my job. (I had taken a leave of absence with the dream of one day returning to the work I loved.) You see, I had been re-ceiving guidance that made no sense to me. Why tell me to quit my job when I couldn't work anyway? Why tell me to leave the E.R. and use my gifts when I wasn't going to live long enough to help anyone? My guidance confused me, yet it was confoundedly consistent.

As I lowered my forehead to the rock, I decided that I would acknowledge my "senseless" guidance, if God would just make it clear to me that it truly *was* guidance. I didn't even nego-tiate with God and say, "Make me healthy and I'll do what you ask." Instead I said, "If this is what you want me to do, then you figure it out. I'm too tired and drained. You work out the de-tails, and I'll show up." I promised that if God gave me a sign, I would listen. I would give up being a nurse in the E.R. It was the first time I had been ready to acknowledge that God might know what he was doing. There was going to be a party in heaven that night.

A party atmosphere seemed to have invaded Peru, too. As I rejoined the group, everyone was smiling at me and seemed ex-cited.

"Look behind you, Christel!"

I turned. A llama was standing just a few feet from me.

The group was ecstatic. "Your spirit guide is here. You've

gotten your sign," they cried.

That llama was the most incredible creature. There was a presence about him, as if he were demanding to be noticed. There was an ethereal quality one could not ignore. The gaze of this llama took me into a moment of stillness that transcended my earthly existence.

But the sense of peace I felt inside was cut short as I came to my senses. Sure, llamas have beautiful and loving eyes. Sure, I was drawn to those eyes. But...

I felt like I had been drawn into a world that was foreign to me. I thought I had a scientific mind that demanded empirical proof – that is, physical proof, something you can see, taste, touch, smell. Empirical proof is the basis for Western medicine. The truth is, what I had was a skeptical mind (okay, perhaps I had a mildly rigid mind, too), and I would not allow myself to be deceived.

"Nope," I shook my head. "This is no sign. Llamas are indigenous to Peru. This one probably escaped from his herder and found the same path we took." My moment of transcendence had passed, and I had clearly disappointed the group. Now they were shaking their heads at me.

Still, I stuck to what my head knew. This llama had wandered away from his flock and coincidentally arrived at the same spot as me. For heaven's sake, llamas are everywhere in Peru!

As we moved on, our shaman guide talked about revitalizing the body through humming certain tones through the stone walls of the roofless enclosure we headed for. As I half-heartedly listened, I wondered what I was doing in the middle of Peru with people with very different beliefs and practices from me, traversing the rocky paths inside Machu Picchu while feeling so unwell. My thoughts were interrupted by an elbow in my ribs. I brought my mind back from its wanderings and noticed that the group had airy smiles of expectancy focused on me again.

"Look down," someone said.

There, carved in a stone sitting on the floor of the enclosure, was the image I had seen in my meditation. I took out my sketch. Sure enough, they were the same. I could feel the group holding its breath. Again, I wanted a sign so badly that I almost gave in.

"No," I said. "This is not a sign. I probably saw the floor of this enclosure on the Discovery Channel or in a National Geographic when I was younger. The image was probably in the back of my brain, and that's how I drew the picture."

Now I had truly disappointed the group. But I had to be sure. I wasn't going to base a life-changing decision on an equivocal sign. As we left the enclosure I asked the shaman who traveled with the group what it was.

"This is the healing temple," he stated simply.

"What is that carved stone on the floor about?"

"That is where they mixed the special herbs for healing," he replied and walked away.

I felt an odd sensation run through me. It felt like I was coming apart at the seams. I was also getting irritable as my orderly and sensible world appeared to be falling down around me. True, all of this magical stuff *seemed* real – but you can't take New York out of a New Yorker, no matter where she is. Then and there I set my intention in stone. I knew what I needed and I wasn't backing down.

"Now listen," I commanded the group. "I need a sign that is so big and so clear, I have no choice but to notice it. It will have to stop me in my tracks." At that moment I remembered the saying, "Be careful what you pray for."

For the rest of the day I had an unsettled feeling. Looking back on it, I realize it was the feeling one gets when life is about to stop making sense or following traditional rules. I know my angels were surrounding me and giggling. I could almost feel their anticipation as they watched a mere mortal human dig in her heels — only to have the ground pulled out from under her. I picture myself with a determined face, holding on to my skepticism, standing on thin air. The look of astonishment as I gaze down at my feet, which are standing on nothing, turns to sheepish laughter when I see my angels are openly guffawing. There is nothing to anchor me, nothing to grab on to; I am in a freefall. I was learning detachment from the physical world, from ego, from my cherished belief that the world is somewhat orderly and follows basic rules. I was also learning that I was not always in charge, and yes, God does work both in mysterious and very obvious — not to mention humorous — ways.

That night we had permission to return to Machu Picchu after hours for a special "releasing" ceremony. I had no idea what I would be releasing. Around midnight we set off through the drizzle and fog to reach our destination. The path was not easy. Climbing among the moss-covered rocks was slippery and dangerous. I had no flashlight and the full moon was obscured. To our left was a sheer rock face and to our right a drop ranging from fifty feet to six thousand feet. After walking for about twenty minutes, feeling soggy and wondering what the heck I was doing out there, the group suddenly stopped in its tracks. I was called forward. Maneuvering through the single line of people, I reached the group leader. She had a mischievous grin and the light of hope in her eyes.

"Do you think this could be your sign?"

Looking past her, I saw three llamas, comfortably nestled across our narrow path. Our Peruvian guides were trying to move them, but they would not budge. All the shouting and shooing and tugging were of no avail. We could go no further.

I did have to laugh. Here were three llamas that not only stopped me in my tracks, but forced me to notice them because the situation was so funny. I walked over to the first llama and looked deeply into his eyes and knew I was talking to my guardian angel. I felt an understanding pass between us.

"I hear you," I said with a nod. "I have my sign. I will quit the E.R. and use my gift full-time." It no longer mattered that I was too ill to work. I simply accepted the guidance God had been trying to give me for so long.

The group sighed in relief until they realized that the three llamas really wouldn't move, and we would have to backtrack along the treacherous path to find an alternate route to our destination. The group was not pleased with me, but I didn't care. I knew that I would be releasing my life as I knew it at our ceremony. It was both frightening and exciting. I felt my angels around me and could do little more than chuckle with them. Paco the llama turned out to be the perfect spirit guide after all. I thanked God for his infinite patience and humor.

I was changed that night. The best way to describe that change is that I became less who I thought I was and more open to who I would become. The struggle inherent in fighting my illness seemed to melt away. The need to understand or explain was of no importance anymore. My fear of the unknown was replaced by an openness to whatever my next adventure would be. I felt soft and malleable, as if I'd been transformed from a concrete human with her heels dug in to an ethereal being of spirit and essence capable of standing on air. I had surrendered and now the Holy Spirit could work through me.

Please don't think that suddenly I was filled with trust and ready to conquer the world. I wasn't. As our trip wore on, I still had questions about the logistical realities of following my guidance. However, that fear was no longer my focus. The need to follow my divine guidance became more important than my fear. This enabled me to take the first step, which is often the hardest part of the journey.

From Machu Picchu we traveled through the countryside to a remote, cobblestoned town called Oyantambo. The snowy Andes glistened like pearls, and our surroundings were tranquil and beautiful. Our Peruvian guides brought us to a tiny village and then up the cliffs to a beautiful meadow. There were even more rocks to climb to reach the temple where we were headed, and three of us opted to stay down below in the valley. I noticed a large rock off to the side and it intrigued me. Our group leader said it was the healing rock. Shamans would put a person on the rock and perform healing rituals.

As the three of us walked toward the rock, seemingly from nowhere, little children appeared in the meadow. They wore ragged and dirty clothing. Their noses ran and their chests heaved with coughing. Some were malnourished. We decided that they were prime candidates for the healing rock.

One by one, we took the children by the hand and had them lie down on the rock. We gently put our hands on them. We sent them love. We envisioned clearing out all negative energies from them. I had learned about this kind of healing during my nursing years when I studied complementary medicine.

Soon these children were laughing and cuddling with us. Their little smiles and bright eyes seemed to light the meadow with enchantment. It was one of the most perfect moments I have ever experienced. There was love and lightness shining from them when they motioned that I should lie on the rock myself and receive some healing.

I lay down and felt their little hands about my body. I remember sensing their innate happiness – so incongruent with their outer appearance. I relaxed into that rock, felt the love of all those children, and didn't question how such great power could emanate from such little beings.

Suddenly I heard flute music and was captivated by the haunting tune. The children turned as the flute player climbed onto the healing rock and looked down at me. I felt a rush of love mingled with sadness. His eyes bore into me as he stood straddling me and opened my heart with the music of his flute. Time stood still as all the sadness, fear, anger, and distrust that I held flowed from me and drained into the rock. I felt paralyzed yet content.

Then the flute quieted. The young man – whom I later learned was a shaman-in-training – bent over me and placed his hands on my head. I felt the power surging into my head – and exploding. I could see millions of tiny bright white stars shooting from his hands. They rushed through my brain, my arms, my legs. In almost the same instant, those stars seemed to light up my entire body. I could feel energy and life surging through my every cell. Then the flutist removed his hands and went back to playing the flute.

He never spoke a word when he left the rock. There were no words that could be spoken, for I knew in that moment that I had been healed from MS. I cannot fully describe the experience – it is too personal and the English language lacks the words to do justice to it – except to say that I was touched by the grace of God.

After I had composed myself, I met up with the rest of the group, who had returned from the temple. I wanted to remember this place of healing, so I asked the shaman who traveled with us where we were.

"Look up and tell me what you see."

I looked up and saw rocks. Peru is filled with rocks. I said so.

"Follow the line of the rocks," he said quietly. "What does it look like?"

I started getting that familiar feeling – like a chill wind – that means something amazing is about to happen to me. I think my angels were riding the chill wind that day, telling me, *Look up, you idiot! What does it look like?* I felt shivers course through my body as I examined the outline of the rocks.

"It looks like an animal," I said.

The shaman was patient, so very patient. "What kind of animal?"

I looked again – and there it was. The rocks and terraces had been carved to form the shape of a sitting llama. My eyes met the shaman's, and he smiled with the wisdom and patience of a true healer.

"What is this place?" I whispered.

"This," he said, turning to take in the exquisite and expansive view, "is the temple of the llama."

❖   ❖   ❖

Synchronicity changed my life to the best it's ever been. I also realized that had I not been estranged from my brother, I wouldn't have gone to Peru. God uses everything and anything to work with us.

Have I learned a few things along the way? Absolutely, and one of those things is to be willing to venture outside the box – the mindset – in which I was raised. When you do, you discover that outside-the-box experiences come to you more and more often. You get to know your own version of the chill wind that signals the moment when the Holy Spirit comes in.

CHAPTER 11

Linking Emotional Patterns
and Specific Diseases

Breast cancer, prostate problems, adult-onset diabetes, and migraine
are usually rooted in a person's toxic beliefs.

During my sixteen years in Emergency Medicine and my decades as a Medical Intuitive, I have learned several valuable lessons:

- Treating the symptoms of disease rarely cures the patient. You have to treat the cause.

- If people get some benefit — emotional, psychological, or practical (like being supported financially) — from their disease, they don't get well no matter what treatment you give them.

- Certain personality traits and personal beliefs are linked with specific diseases.

This chapter focuses on the last of these lessons, and the four diseases I want to talk to you about are ones that are plaguing our Western culture: breast cancer, prostate cancer, adult-onset diabetes, and migraines.

Before I proceed, however, I want to offer a caution. At the beginning of this book, I talked about the perils of recipe medicine, which assumes that everyone with symptom "X" has disease "Y." I also noted that this tendency to use generalizations to diagnose illness has spread to my own field.

Here's the bottom line: No one can tell you for certain that a particular symptom you have is rooted in a particular belief or behavior of yours unless they have read your energy field and seen the link. For example, if you have a problem with your legs, it could be emotionally linked to a fear of moving forward, as many alternative practitioners would likely tell you, or it could be an anatomical deficit that's causing your pain. But it could just as easily be linked to not standing up for yourself. Or it could also be caused by feeling unsafe in your home. (This fear is often present in people with varicose veins or thrombophlebitis (a clot in a leg vein). That's because your legs are connected to your root chakra, which is about safety and survival. If you are feeling unsafe, your root chakra gets blocked, and energy does not flow freely to your legs. This impairs their health.

Also, there's a difference between having pain in your legs and having a particular disease. Each disease has its own unique vibration or energetic signature. But all diseases have a low vibration, which can resonate with a low vibration in you caused by things that drain your energy, like tribal beliefs.

There are, however, certain beliefs and behaviors that *usually* correlate with certain diseases. I want to tell you about them. I am trusting you not to apply these descriptions wholesale to your own situation. Think about them. Look into your heart.

Ask your soul. See if they fit for you. If so, you may be at risk.

Breast Cancer

Martha, thirty-nine, was vibrant and energetic. She appeared very happy. Newly remarried, she was excited to be a wife after raising her ten-year-old son by herself. But when she sat down in my office I noted some fear in her first chakra. I was puzzled because being newly married should have made her feel more secure, not less.

Martha told me she had been diagnosed with breast cancer. She wanted to know if there was anything I could do to help her. I began by scanning her energy field, in which I saw a running "video" of her life up to the present day, as well as her beliefs, her patterns of behavior, and her physical condition. Here's what I saw.

When Martha was eighteen, her mother died of cancer. Her mom's last six months had been very, very hard on the family. After the funeral, Martha's dad said to her, "You are the only family I have now. We must stick together. If I lose you too, I'll die." Martha was about to go away to college, and struggled over whether to go or stay home. In the end, she decided to go.

Two years later, when Martha's father remarried and moved away, she felt like she'd failed him by neglecting to keep the family together. She hadn't tried hard enough, she thought: She'd been selfish and gone to college instead. Her self-esteem plunged.

At school, Martha fell into a pattern of doing things for others and not taking care of herself. Her goal was never to fail her new "family" of college friends, and she worked tirelessly to keep everyone happy. She neglected herself and didn't speak up for her needs. Her lack of self-esteem made it difficult for her to receive without reciprocating. She became the consummate giver and caretaker.

Because she missed the nurturing presence of her mother, Martha sought boyfriends at college who would play that role for her. When she discovered she was pregnant, she decided to have an abortion. She never told her father and never forgave herself. After graduating, Martha married and continued to be a consummate caretaker. She simply did whatever it took to keep her family together and happy.

When my scan was complete, Martha said, "I know your emotions can affect why we get sick, but I don't understand why I have breast cancer. I have such a big heart, I am so loving with others. It doesn't make sense."

"Okay," I said, "let's start with a rundown of the main emotional traits I have seen in women who get breast cancer. First, their relationships revolve around taking care of others, often to the exclusion of taking care of themselves. They have a tribal belief that caretaking is their job and they're not good wives, mothers, or friends unless they are constantly concerned with the welfare of others.

"They don't know how to nurture themselves or speak up for their own needs. They are uncomfortable receiving because they don't feel they're worth it. They avoid confrontation. They manipulate or compromise instead, even if it's not in their best interests. They think they do it because they want to keep the peace or don't want to hurt anyone's feelings – but it's really because they don't think their needs or wants are important."

Martha looked dumbstruck.

"There's one more important thing," I said. "I have found that women with breast cancer almost always have a secret, something they can't forgive themselves for. This lack of forgiveness lowers their vibration and shuts down the energy flowing to their heart chakra. And the heart chakra, of course, is located near the breasts. In addition, having a guilty secret makes them feel ashamed and gives them a vague sense of owing a debt. It makes them think that they don't deserve to be happy, to have a good marriage or an easy path in life. The fallout from their guilty secret pervades their entire lives."

At this point I stopped talking and watched Martha take it all in. She admitted that she fit the breast-cancer profile. But she said she didn't want to change. Caring for others was the right way to live, she told me. It was what made life worthwhile.

As I closed the door behind her, I remembered that Martha had come to ask *why* she had breast cancer – not how to heal it. Sadly, she had gotten just what she came for.

◆　◆　◆

When I worked with Nancy, a fifty-two-year-old account-ant, the situation was totally different. Nancy was receiving chemo for breast cancer when I did her reading. I saw that she was not speaking to her mother, and this was causing her tre-mendous distress. I talked with Nancy about the energetic com-ponents of breast cancer, as I had with Martha, and she, too, quickly recognized herself. But in Nancy's case, she was deter-mined to make whatever changes were necessary to heal. She left ready to call her mother and mend their rift. Now, with her breast cancer – and her nonstop caregiving – five years behind her, Nancy is the happiest she's ever been.

◆　◆　◆

Breast cancer is so prevalent nowadays, we have to get more aggressive toward healing it. I think that understanding the emo-tional patterns that are linked to breast cancer is one of the key steps.

I ask my clients with breast cancer to take this self-quiz. Try it. See if you recognize yourself or someone you care about. If so, you (or she) can begin to make different choices that can lead to preventing or healing breast cancer.

1. Can I accept a compliment without looking away or denying it?

2. When a friend buys me dinner, do I simply say, "Thank you," or do I insist, "I'll buy next time"?

3. Do I take care of myself?

4. Do I nap when my body is tired?

5. Can I say no when I don't want to do something?

6. Do I blame myself for something like the breakup of my marriage?

7. Can I forgive myself when I act human?

8. Have I lost sight of myself and my personal goals in my marriage, work, or personal relationships?

9. Am I living only for other people: my husband, my kids, or my parents?

10. Do people rely on me as the strong one? Am I uncomfortable sharing my problems with others for fear of bothering them or because my problems might burden or sadden them?

11. Can I honestly say I am happy as things are? If not, do I avoid doing anything about it?

12. Is keeping my family together at all costs my primary goal in life?

13. Do I have a secret that causes tremendous guilt and

shame? Do I live in fear that I will be judged for it? Is it eating away at me?

Prostate Problems

Scott is forty-two, and he's a delight to be with. Women find him sexy and articulate. They also feel safe with him. He is playful, loving, and honest to a fault. Scott's physique is extraordinary — he could do one of those Pepsi commercials where all the women run to the window to look at him. Unfortunately, Scott didn't know any of this.

Scott came for a reading because for the first time in his life, he was sick and in pain. To others this was shocking because he looked so healthy. Numerous tests later, no definitive diagnosis had been reached. Thus, a professed skeptic and proud of it, Scott came to me.

During his reading, I noted two important tribal beliefs that were unconsciously driving Scott's life. First, *It is important to treat a woman well and sex is how you show her you love her.* Second, *A man without money isn't a man at all — if he can't take care of his family, he's a failure. Having money means you're powerful.* These tribal beliefs had deeply affected Scott's second chakra, where issues about money, creativity, and sexuality reside. The second chakra also rules the sexual organs, so when that chakra becomes blocked, the sexual organs suffer.

I also read in Scott's energy field the history of how his tribal beliefs had come to affect his health. One morning he had awakened with a painful inflammation of his prostate gland and couldn't make love to his wife. They abstained for over three weeks while the swelling subsided, and Scott silently berated himself for his loss of manhood. Finally the big day arrived and Scott was well again. He started to make love to his wife — but he couldn't sustain an erection.

At that point, Scott's whole world caved in. All of a sudden he was a bad husband (in his estimation), a judgment which was based on his tribal beliefs. Then, a month later, he was laid off from his job. Now Scott thought he was not only a bad husband but a failure to boot. According to his tribal beliefs, he had ceased being a good and powerful man.

These two events had been enough to tip the scales in Scott's already ailing second chakra. His vibration dropped; prostate cancer grew in his body and progressed rapidly. Although Scott was still unaware of his diagnosis, his tribal beliefs would trap him into believing that death was a better alternative than living as a failure.

I referred to Scott's second chakra as "already ailing" because his problems began long before his prostate started to hurt. When Scott was sixteen, his family hit rough financial times, and his tribal beliefs rose up to shame him. He became embarrassed at his cheap clothing and his family's straitened lifestyle. When his father confessed that he no longer felt "like a real man," Scott swore that he would die before he would allow himself to fail as a man or as a husband.

This vow set off an internal energetic reaction: Scott constantly worried about money and his ability to perform sexually. He was in a constant state of fight or flight, which lowered his vibration and began to wear down his body.

When a fellow high-school student made a joke about his homemade lunch, calling it a "welfare meal," Scott was deeply wounded. He didn't feel powerful or manly, and his self-esteem plummeted. He became unable to accept compliments or acknowledge his strengths and talents. This continued into his adult life. To Scott, the fact that he was honest, loving, compassionate, and a good listener meant nothing. It was only his ability to earn plenty of money and be a good (i.e., sexually active) husband that counted.

Scott pushed himself for years, unrelenting in his quest for success. Unfortunately, his path was blocked by other tribal beliefs that also affected his second chakra. These were *Money doesn't come easily, you must work hard for it,* and *There's never enough money.*

So Scott was caught between a rock and hard place – which is the only reason he came to me. Ironically, his goal was to get well so he could go back to work (where he would proceed to work himself to death). As we talked, I discovered Scott was so invested in his tribal beliefs that he couldn't let them go. Since there was no healing for him that way, he asked me to do a laying on of hands to heal him. I refused. There was no way I would contribute to Scott's death by making him well enough to work himself into an early grave.

Next Scott asked me for a sample of my work, hoping to negotiate my acquiescence. I saw right through him, but I thought it was worth a shot, so I raised his vibration.

Scott was silent, then tears filled his eyes. He looked up at me in wonder and said, "I felt like I was free, like I was twenty years old. I had no tension. I felt wonderful."

The feeling lasted about fifteen minutes. Then Scott asked me again to do a laying on of hands. I explained that any healing I did would be temporary unless he changed his tribal beliefs and raised his vibration so it no longer resonated with prostate cancer. Any healing I did wouldn't last because his vibration would just drop again.

"But I can't change! It's too hard!" he exclaimed. "I am who I am."

Here was evidence of another tribal belief blocking Scott's way: *Change is hard.* I asked Scott to start working on the tribal beliefs in his root chakra. I explained how tribal beliefs can stand in the way of healing, and I gave him instructions on how to change them. But he wasn't interested. For him, it was more important to honor his tribe — and the beliefs he inherited from them — than to get well.

Adult-Onset Diabetes

David was fifty-one, but he looked sixty-five. He came to see me because he had just been diagnosed with diabetes. What I saw before me was a man who was totally lacking in passion. When I did a reading for him, I saw he was trapped in a loveless marriage. David was the sole support for his wife and three children. He went to work each day, and knew there would be no respite no matter how weary he was. He had to take care of his family because that, he told me, is what a good father does.

Feeling you are in a situation with no way out is one of the key traits in people who develop diabetes as adults. Another trait is sacrificing your dream.

Imagine being young and energetic. You want to make a difference in the world. You dream of working for conservation; you want to help protect the whales. Or perhaps you dream of owning a small cabin deep in the tranquil woods where you can meditate and photograph wildlife. Or you may simply be unhappy in your marriage and dream of finding your true soulmate.

But life always seems to get in the way of achieving your dream. You invest your energy in situations that drain you instead of energize you. You tell yourself you just need to keep doing "X" for five more years and then you can retire, or build that cabin, or leave your marriage. But five more years come and go, and still you are going through the motions of life, feeling more and more trapped in your unhappy, energy-draining situation.

Then you wake up one morning and discover that you've given up on your dream.

Resignation seems to drip from your pores. Life has become an obligation, a duty, rather than something fun or exciting. There are so many "musts" in your life that there's no room for your wants. Your desire for happiness withers; "I do what I have to do" becomes your motto. Putting one foot in front of another is the best you hope for. Life is a chore. Your third chakra — where self-esteem, courage, and confidence reside — becomes blocked.

In all the adult-onset diabetics I have worked with, I see the same thing: no energy is flowing through their third chakra. These clients have no relationship with themselves. They do no nurturing or caretaking of themselves. They are driven by and locked into old tribal beliefs about hard work, duty, and obligation. They tell themselves, *This is life, so just get on with it.* They feel trapped. They get little pleasure out of life. When you add to this the fact that because they are diabetic, they must deny themselves the pleasure of eating certain foods, their "celibate" lifestyle is complete: little or no fun, few "sweet" moments, and a lot of hard work.

My first question for someone like this is always, "What was your dream?" Some can remember it. Some say they never had one. Some say they had one but can't even remember what it was. Healing for people with adult-onset diabetes depends on their reviving their dreams and allowing themselves to achieve them. Then they can really *live*, not merely exist trapped in a situation with no way out.

Migraines

Cynthia, a hair stylist with her own shop, appears very successful. She's thirty-one, single, funny, and loving – and she suf-ferers nearly incessant migraines. She came to see me because her headaches had become so frequent that they threatened her livelihood.

During my reading of Cynthia, I saw an energetic ball of chaos swirling around her head. It was like watching the light show at Epcot Center. Like Cynthia, most migraine sufferers ex-perience a high level of chaos. This can take the form of "head chatter," or it may be manifested in the external events of their lives. They are frequently in a mild state of fight or flight.

Because Cynthia's thoughts were moving faster than the Tasmanian devil whirling around and kicking up dust, it was dif-ficult to do a reading, so I did some chakra balancing on her, then took another look.

Cynthia's first chakra was shut down. She was disconnected from her family of origin, and this was bringing up serious sur-vival issues for her. Cynthia had no safety net if her business failed. She had nowhere to turn if she needed help. The running video I saw of her childhood revealed an absent father who had left when Cynthia was eight. After that, money was desperately scarce, and her mother paraded one "scary" boyfriend after an-other through their home in hopes of finding another husband. When Cynthia tried to tell her mom that she was really afraid of one of these men (and for good reason – the man had molested her), her mother made her choice clear: The boyfriend was more important than Cynthia. (Needless to say, this incident caused problems for Cynthia in addition to the migraines, but it wasn't the priority for this reading.)

The wound caused by her mother's choice was enough to shut down Cynthia's root chakra. Without her mother's protec-tion, she wasn't safe. The incident also taught her she couldn't trust people, and she couldn't count on anyone. The chaos in

Cynthia's head was her way of avoiding the reality that her mother hadn't given her the protection or nurturing she needed. The pain she felt about this abandonment was so immense that she had to live in her head so as not to feel it.

The key to healing Cynthia's migraines was to open up her root chakra and create a feeling of safety in her life, thus calming the fight-or-flight response that she lived with. Cynthia worked diligently for two months examining the tribal beliefs that didn't serve her highest good, using deep breathing and conscious relaxation to ease her anxiety, doing short-term meditation and trauma-release work, and receiving chakra balancing. I taught her how to communicate deeply and honestly with her friends. She learned she could count on them and they would be there for her. Cynthia also ended her relationship with a boyfriend who kept her on edge – in a constant but unconscious state of fight-or-flight – and learned how to forgive her mother for not protecting her when she was young.

At the end of that time, Cynthia said she felt like a new person. What was actually happening was that she was becoming acquainted with the wonderful child she had been, the child she had lost touch with at age eight. Her migraines stopped completely. Cynthia is now able to provide comfort and security for herself as well as to accept love, protection, and nurturing from others. She is also happily married!

CHAPTER 12

Going Beyond Illness

We have the power to heal...

In recent years I have started working more and more with clients who are not physically ill but, despite outward signs of success, feel there is something missing in their lives. Maybe they are emotionally stuck or feel their life has gotten off course. Maybe they can't find the right person, or they are failing in business. Or maybe they have only a vague sense that being alive doesn't feel as good as it should.

How can a Medical Intuitive help someone with a non-medical problem? Because happiness in all aspects of your life depends entirely upon having a lot of energy flowing through you. This can happen only when you resolve your conflicts and embrace your shadow. Blocked chakras, low vibration, and tribal beliefs can open a direct line to maladies in your life as well as your physical body. Unhappiness *in whatever form it takes* is a message that you are out of the **flow**, out of alignment with your soul, and hence with God.

By the same token, when I talk about healing, I don't mean healing only physical illness and distress. I mean healing whatever takes you out of the flow and away from the deep and joyful life your soul desires for you. Your soul always knows what's best for you because it is connected to your Higher Power.

For many people, developing an illness is a wakeup call, the first indication that they are severely out of flow. (There are a number of things to be learned from getting ill, but first and foremost it is an indication that something is out of balance.) For others the first indication they are out of flow is that something they want very badly is eluding them, and they don't know why. It may be a happy relationship, financial success, or peace of mind.

I work with many clients who have issues like these – and more. Some people want to stop repetitive patterns that aren't good for them. Others want to know what they should do with their lives or wonder which decision is the right one to make.

Flow

The state of serenity you feel when your heart, mind, and actions are in harmony with God's highest desire for you. People usually think of flow as a state when external things are going well. But flow is really about internal things going well. It's this internal state that smoothes the way for external success.

Some simply come to see me because their lives feel so hard and they don't know what to do about it. Many come because they have a spiritual longing, and they don't know how to connect with God. They want to learn how to hear guidance and feel God's love. All of these are examples of being out of flow.

Being out of the flow is what happens when you are not saying, thinking, or living in harmony with your soul's desire.

Being in the flow is when your ego

is out of the way. You are listening to your guidance cleanly, without trying to get a certain answer. Your behavior is aligned with your soul's desire for you: You are not caretaking others. Your life still has bumps, but your response to them is very different. You don't have to worry about how to handle things until your head explodes. The answers are within you.

For example, you can listen inside to see if you are in the flow. Maybe you are saying, "I want to see my family for the holidays," when you have no magnetics for doing that but feel you should go anyway. One clue is when there is too much discussion in your head about something, too much chatter, instead of a silent knowing. All that ego-based head chatter drowns out the voice of your Higher Power. Besides, it's tiring!

Being in the flow is being honest with others, not trying to manipulate them into liking you or caretaking them so they won't leave you. It's getting out of a toxic relationship even though you are scared to be alone. It's being in the present with what is instead of worrying about the future or feeling guilty about the past.

Being in the flow is knowing who you are and living with profound honesty and deep integrity.

◆　◆　◆

Carey was fifty-four. He came to see me because he was bored with his life. He was wealthy, owned several race horses and a number of fancy cars, hung out with the rich and famous, and was tall, dark, and handsome to boot. He seemed to have it all.

Carey heard that I was able to "see" a person's true essence, and he wanted to know what his purpose was here on the earth. He was hoping his life would add up to more than financial success and luxurious possessions.

This kind of reading is fun for me. I look forward in time and see the results of particular choices that mean the difference between boredom (which is a lack of magnetics) and getting on one's true path and really living. It's fun because I get to see another person become who he really is, do what truly brings him joy, and live with a passion that knocks his socks off! It's my idea of being alive.

Carey sat down, self-assured, confident, and perhaps a tad skeptical. But, as he put it, it was only money he was risking in consulting me, so what the heck.

Carey was used to being around movers and shakers, so I shook him. "Carey, I am going to give it to you in a nutshell. What I call the New York version."

He smiled, and later confided he was pleased I didn't go into a psychic trance, moan, and mumble vague predictions.

"If you don't sell your business immediately," I said, commanding all of his attention — mind, heart, and soul — "you will have a heart attack within six months."

I leaned back in my chair and watched him. Carey never blinked, balked at the information, or asked if I was certain. He simply nodded.

"I believe you," he said quietly. "My father died of a heart attack at fifty-five, and my brother died of a heart attack at fifty-four. I had a feeling."

Then his brain pushed his soul out of the way and took over.

"But I can't sell my business! I'd take a tremendous beating. The market is down. How will I live without the income it produces?" He continued in this vein for several minutes.

"You'll make it work, or you'll die," I replied. "Your heart chakra* is closed, and this has had an effect on your heart muscle. There is a fair amount of blockage. I want you to go for a cardiac catheterization. Medication will also be very beneficial until you turn this around."

"You mean, I won't die at fifty-five?"

"Not of a heart attack," I smiled.

Carey came to see me for seven more sessions. I helped him work out the logistics of letting go of his business by using intuitive information for problem-solving and decision-making. I taught him to access that kind of information in himself. The key for him was to choose to let go of the life he was leading. It took Carey three days to make the announcement to his employees, and almost five months to literally dump the business, get rid of the horses and cars, and shuck his extravagant lifestyle. The less he had, the happier he became.

On the fifth session I asked Carey if he was ready to know why he was here on earth. He was. I described the pictures I saw in my mind: He was talking to very unloved, angry, and lonely children. He was involved in creating intimacy, safety, and bonding – something that had eluded him for most of his life.

I can't tell you the name of the organization he started because that would break confidence by revealing his true identity. Suffice to say it is very large, and it involves educating and loving inner-city children who would otherwise be in gangs, on the street, or dead before they're eighteen.

Carey not only used his old connections to raise money and get the organization going, he now spends one-on-one time with the children. He's having a blast. He is living his life's purpose, he loves making a difference, and he's healthy. His old life of par-

---

* Also known as the fourth chakra. In it resides your ability to feel, to love, and to hurt. It's where we hold attachments to others, and it is affected by our ability to forgive ourselves and others.

ties, fundraisers, back-scratching politics, being seen, and keeping up an image is like a vague memory. And yes, he passed his fifty-fifth birthday. It was one of the happiest he's ever had.

◆　◆　◆

Will is a quiet and sensitive guy. He worked hard and earned good money, started his own company and did even better. At fifty-two he had enough to retire comfortably with his wife. Unfortunately, he was bound by tribal beliefs about being happy. His family of origin had struggled financially and taught him that this was how things were. Will felt guilty about his good fortune and his easy life.

In his reading, I noticed that Will had no magnetics for the work he was doing. In fact, it was severely draining his energy and causing a spiritual depression. His doctor had diagnosed him with clinical depression and put him on antidepressants to increase his serotonin level, but they weren't working. I wasn't surprised. Spiritual depression is when you go against your soul and ignore your intuition – that is, your guidance. Antidepressants won't help because there's nothing wrong with your serotonin level.

Will hated confrontation and found it easier to acquiesce to his family and their beliefs than stand up for himself. He also had a tribal belief that being sensitive – which he was – wasn't manly.

We talked about letting go of the tribal beliefs that bound him, and as he relaxed into the session, I saw a wonderful image, which I shared with him.

"Will, this is what I see. You are on an island or in an island-type environment with palm trees and flowers and surf. You are wearing one of those flowery shirts, and stubble has grown on your face. In fact, your shorts are cutoffs, and you are walking along the edge of the water. You stop, sit down and close your eyes, and ..."

I had to stop and laugh. I shook my head. "Will, this is crazy, but it looks like one of those advertisements for stress-free living – complete with yoga classes and meditation. Sorry it sounds so stereotypical, but it's what I see. You are the yoga instructor and you're leading a group through its paces on the sand."

Will stared at me open-mouthed. Tears started running down his face. At that moment he didn't care if I saw him being sensitive. He exhaled, then swallowed and tried to speak.

"It's my dream," he said quietly. "It's what I've always wanted – to live in the islands and teach yoga. To live in a house on the beach. I've been secretly studying yoga for more than twelve years, and my wife and I have bought some property in Hawaii for a yoga school."

"FANTASTIC!" I hollered. "We're both on the same page! Now let's talk about how to achieve your dream."

I taught Will how to let go of his tribal beliefs: *It's not okay to be happy when your family is struggling, it's not okay for a man to be sensitive,* and *a man has to work to be a good person.* We then worked on building up his second chakra (the seat of our relationship with significant others and our desire to have them love us) so he would no longer sacrifice his dreams in order to please his family. Will learned to take care of himself in addition to taking care of his family. We also worked on his third chakra, where self-esteem, confidence, and courage reside. Will learned to accept his gifts and talents and give up guilt for having an easy life.

That same day Will went home and told his wife he was referring all new business to his competitors. He was ready to start living. Even though he was scared of making some of the changes, he went ahead and did it anyway.

As it turned out, all Will needed was confirmation that the guidance he had been receiving – *Quit your job and live on the beach*

– was genuine. In a few more sessions, we got the logistics worked out, and *voilà!*

Is Will happy in the islands? Did he turn out to be a great yoga instructor? Has he stopped taking his antidepressants and become someone who loves life?

The answer is yes, yes, yes, yes!

CHAPTER 13

The Lowest Vibration of All

When God feels far away, guess who moved?

IF I WERE TO READ your energetic blueprint, the most important thing I would look for is the quality of your connection with your Higher Power: Do you believe God or a Higher Power exists? Do you trust it? Can you hear divine guidance? Michelangelo could. It's what inspired him to paint the Sistine chapel. Is your relationship with your Higher Power in your head or is it in your heart, where it belongs?

Why does the strength – or weakness – of this connection matter? Because having a strong connection with God means we are in touch with our creator – the source of unconditional love, the source of our inspiration, and the source of our guidance, which supports our highest good and makes our life flow. On the other hand, spiritual disconnection shuts off the life force and dramatically lowers your vibration. It is the worst disease on the planet because we can live with an illness or without a limb, but we cannot live without the true source of unconditional love, light, and high vibration: God.

❖

Signs of Spiritual Disconnection

◆ You feel sluggish – life is okay, but nothing special. Things that used to wow you, don't. You feel tired, empty. You start to wonder, is this all there is?

◆ You feel lonely. Even if you are going to work and socializing, you feel deeply alone.

◆ You feel adrift. You have no sense of direction in life.

◆ You question everything, or you question nothing because you lack the energy.

◆ Your inspiration and good ideas have dried up.

◆ You don't say prayers, and you rarely express gratitude for all that you have in your life.

◆ You feel separated from yourself because you can't access your soul.

◆ You can't tell if you've heard guidance or your own thoughts.

◆ You are more involved with yourself and what you want than with God and what God wants for you.

I can see the quality of your relationship with God by looking at the health of your seventh, or crown chakra, which is at the top of your head. The crown chakra is where our spiritual connection resides. I see it as a door that is either wide open, open just a crack, or slammed shut. A wide-open door means the person has a strong connection with God. She is able to hear guidance and feels connected to a greater whole. Creative ideas flow freely and inspiration is routine. She feels safe and loved. Her life is filled with joy.

When the door in someone's crown chakra is partially open – often it's just a crack – the person has a polite indifference to God. This means that when something goes wrong in her life, she prays, bargains, and negotiates with God until all is well again. Then prayer is forgotten or put far down on his "To Do" list.

Generally, someone with a partially open door in his crown chakra isn't completely disconnected spiritually. He may acknowledge there is a God or Higher Power, but he isn't sure if God listens to him. He doesn't trust God. He asks for guidance, but with limitations, just as I used

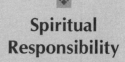

Spiritual Responsibility

Taking responsibility for your life, no matter what illness, wounds, or problems you have and no matter who or what caused them. Being spiritually responsible is the polar opposite of identifying yourself as a victim.

to do. He wants it how he wants it — which essentially means, he doesn't want it. He doesn't trust God to have his best interests at heart.

Trying to negotiate with or manipulate God saps energy from his second chakra and lowers his vibration. Anger and resentment — "How could God let this happen to me/others/the world?" — also lower his vibration.

It seems odd that someone would be afraid to trust in God when intellectually we know that God is good, not evil. But our tribal beliefs almost always override our reason. I worked with a woman named Kathy on restoring her spiritual connection. I guided her to reestablish a relationship with God, and I told her I thought she could reach a new level of **spiritual responsibility**: to dedicate herself to be of service to God and those around her.

Kathy looked both startled and tense as she exclaimed, "I can't do that!"

"Why? What are you afraid of?" I asked.

With complete sincerity, Kathy replied, "If I give my life

over to God, I'll be asked to be a missionary or something. I could end up cleaning toilets in the wilds of Rwanda," she wailed.

I hesitated a moment, then replied, "Kathy, they don't *have* toilets in the wilds of Rwanda!"

Both of us burst out laughing.

In reality, though, tribal beliefs are no laughing matter. They are powerful. Kathy had a tribal belief that being of service to God means hardship: being a missionary, being penniless, being single, being alone. The belief that being of service requires some horrible sacrifice on our parts is extremely common. People have learned to fear God, and fear makes it difficult to trust. Is it any wonder so many people today are in varying stages of spiritual disconnection?

Later I told Kathy about two wonderful people I know who pray daily for God to call them to be missionaries. My point was, there are people who actually want this, so why would God have us do something we didn't enjoy? To torture us? So we can struggle and suffer?

That's another one of those pesky tribal beliefs. You have to remember that religion is humanity's attempt to reach God – and humans wrote many of the rules, which is where these unfounded tribal beliefs come from. I find it ironic that the door in many people's crown chakra can't be completely open to God because of their religious beliefs. Sometimes a person whose crown chakra is open just a crack is not sure whether there is a God or not. She prays occasionally, just in case, but she rarely prays for guidance. If she does, though, and she hears a response, she isn't sure what she's hearing. Is it God or just a voice in her head? With her crown chakra barely open, she doesn't get lots of ideas or inspiration. She tends to feel lost, alone, and lonely.

◆ ◆ ◆

Now let's look at people whose door is slammed shut. There are usually two reasons for this: Either they feel God has failed them at some point (when an abused child's prayer for help isn't answered, for example), or they've never had an experience of a Higher Power because they are agnostic or atheistic, and were raised to rely only on themselves.

Ideas rarely come to someone like this. Inspiration is nil. She feels alone and bereft, like she is floating way out in space on a tether that could break at any moment. She does not communicate with God other than to lash out in anger. Energetically her system is shut down. It's as if she's downstream from a big dam: No water (ideas) flow to her and eventually the river (creativity) dries up. Humans are energetic beings. Cut off that energy and we begin to fade. After a time we become parched and lifeless. The creative spirit dries up.

When I look to see how someone's energetic "dam" began, I see she has gone through something similar to the five stages of dying identified by Elisabeth Kubler-Ross. At first she is shocked that God has apparently abandoned her. Maybe something very painful has happened to her or God hasn't answered her prayers. Next comes anger at being abandoned. Then she tries bargaining. Well, bargaining with God *never* works, so she concludes that God does not exist.

Now things go from bad to worse because she enters the stage of spiritual depression. This is a terrible disease. People with spiritual depression look like the walking dead. They go through the motions of life. They are emotionally flat and have no real dreams, desires, or joy. Life looks gray to them, and their energy fields look gray to me. I see no color or vibrancy or movement in them.

When a person has no connection to Spirit, the world ceases

to make sense. Life becomes meaningless. She feels bereft and powerless. She sees the world as a burned-out, empty place where smoking rubble covers every inch of the once green earth. She is just waiting for her body to die. Her spirit already has.

I call this state energetic suicide, and it happens when all your chakras shut down. It's no fun – and it's deadly. I'll talk more about it later in this chapter.

If you close the door to your source of light, love, inspiration, ideas, feelings, safety, and joy, what is left? A feeling of emptiness – and the complete mess you make of your life because you can't hear guidance. Without a Higher Power to nudge you in the right direction, you will make poor choices about your mate, your work, and your life.

The problem is, you may not know that you have closed the door on God. You may think it's God's fault that you cannot hear guidance. A common thing I hear is: "I *do* pray, but I don't get an answer." What's happening in this case is that you are not praying sincerely. Some part of you is afraid of the answer you might get.

For me, living in a world without God would be dark, bleak, empty, and very, very lonely. We are beings of light, and we are meant to return to that light. Some religions teach that we are born in darkness, sin, and evil. I disagree. Separation from God is the only route to darkness. The more separate you become, the less you notice the light, and the less light shines from within you. The less you shine, the lower and denser your vibration becomes. Do you see now why it's so important for us to shine our brightest? It's our way back home, to the source, to God, to light.*

---

* The process I have developed to reopen the crown chakra and get energy flowing through all the chakras again is called LUMOS™, which is the Latin

The good news about people whose crown chakra is closed is that although they may have reached the stage of depression about God not being there, few have reached the fifth stage of accepting there is no God. A tiny part of them still hopes there is a God and that God cares about them.

Spiritual disconnection doesn't always show on the outside. You may still laugh, play, and interact with others, but not at a deep level. You live with a very low vibration and risk energetic suicide — when all seven of your chakras shut down, and no energy flows through them. No amount of earthly money, love, or psychotherapy can cure spiritual disconnection. Turning toward your Higher Power is the only cure and it helps to have a guide.

◆　◆　◆

Carol, thirty-five, is a sweet and vivacious woman with a quick smile and a slightly mischievous side. By the time she came in for a reading, she was terribly fatigued, had difficulty with her memory, and had been diagnosed with chronic fatigue syndrome. When I did a scan, I had difficulty finding Carol's unique energetic signature at first because her vibration was so low.

When Carol was eight, her father told her she was useless because she wasn't a son. He repeatedly let her know that it was only by "the grace of God" that she was allowed to live in his family. Soon her two brothers joined in taunting her. The scene that unfolded was like something from Cinderella: Carol was responsible for cleaning the house and keeping her brothers happy, and was the butt of many jokes.

---

word for light. The letters also stand for "Lighting the Unconscious Masking of Source." I chose this name because the light is so desperately needed in people with no connection to God. They are dark, as is their world. I teach the LUMOS™ technique so people can raise own their vibrations and let go of their separation from God.

By the age of thirteen, she was fully convinced that she was worthless. At fourteen, when one of her brothers molested her, Carol completely shut down her feelings. She survived by taking care of the family's needs on the assumption that they would cast her out if she stopped.

Carol's pain was immense – too immense for a fourteen-year-old. One night she tried to kill herself. She swallowed a whole bottle of aspirin and went to sleep. Luckily, she vomited much of the aspirin. She also had to go through several grueling hours of hallucinations and severe ringing in her ears. Her family's response to her cry for help was to get angry. Not even fifteen yet, Carol felt trapped and worthless. She fervently wished for death to take her.

As she cried out to God for help one night, her abusive brother overheard her and set her straight. "There is no God," he sneered, "especially not for people like you."

These words sealed Carol's fate. They were like a knife wound to her heart – and to her energy field. The only thing that had kept Carol alive was praying to God for help. Now she knew her prayers fell on deaf ears. This was the moment when her illness began.

They say that sticks and stones can break your bones but words can never hurt you. It's not true. Words can have a lasting and truly harmful effect on your chakra system, especially when you already lack self-esteem, give your power away to others, or have been taught to never buck authority. Carol lost all hope. She never prayed again. She believed there was nothing and no one who would ever help her.

When Carol turned her back on God, she shut down her crown chakra and her life force began to fade. She was resigned to leading a lonely and joyless life. Even though her soul – that small, often-discounted voice deep inside of each of us – shouted to her that her family was toxic and she should move far away, she was too depleted and scared to try. In her mind, the only way to escape her misery was to die. Death equaled freedom.

Our thoughts and beliefs are *so* powerful. Carol's belief that God would not help her was self-fulfilling. It caused her crown chakra to shut down. It prevented her from hearing guidance, and feeling love, safety, and a connection to a presence outside herself.

Carol continued to live as her family's caretaker until she could no longer function physically. It was this illness, diagnosed as chronic fatigue syndrome, that brought her to see me.

In our first session, I saw the vibration of lupus, not chronic fatigue. Lupus is a chronic disease that affects the skin, joints, blood, and kidneys. It causes inflammation, tissue damage, and pain. An autoimmune disorder, it stimulates the body to make antibodies directed against itself. For most people, lupus is a mild disease affecting only a few organs, but for Carol it was a serious and even life-threatening problem. This was no time to talk about Carol's childhood or work on building her self-esteem. A person can survive a terrible childhood. A person can even survive without self-esteem. But what I have seen consistently in my work as a Medical Intuitive is that you cannot survive without a connection to a higher power in some form or another.

So I sat down and prayed with Carol. I helped her get past her misconceptions about God and began using LUMOS™ with her. I showed her how to reopen her crown chakra. Most important, I taught her that she wasn't alone, that God really was there for her. All she had to do was keep the lines of communication open.

It made all the difference in her healing. She was able to tap into her guidance, which relieved her anxiety at feeling unloved and alone, and stopped her from feeling trapped. Carol's life went from unbearable to joyous as she learned to feel God's presence. Opening her crown chakra opened the flow of energy to the rest of her system and raised her vibration. She felt inspired to live and be of service to others. For the first time in her life, Carol felt safe. She wanted to live! She moved far away from her family, and to this day her blood markers continue to test negative for *any* autoimmune disease.

◆ ◆ ◆

Joan, fifty-four, lived in the doctor's office. Very much the victim, she came to me not to get well, but to understand why she was plagued with poor health. It was the classic "Poor me!" approach. She had no energy and felt depressed sometimes; none of her "stupid doctors" could give her a diagnosis.

Joan felt disconnected from her husband, her tribe of origin, and from people as a whole. Her present was spent predominantly in the past, where she relived the few real wounds of her childhood – and all the perceived wounds. At least sixty percent of her energy was devoted to the past.

As a child, Joan had been taught, as Karl Marx put it, that "religion is the opiate of the masses," and God only helps good people. Her tribal belief was, *When something bad happens to people, it's because they did something wrong.* For the past five

Archetype

A predisposition to act and react in a certain way. For instance, when someone with a predominant Detective archetype encounters a child crying over a broken toy, she would say, "How did that toy break?" Someone with a predominant Mother archetype would bend down and comfort the child. The gods and goddesses of ancient myths were personifications of archetypes. Some examples are Venus, who personified the Lover; Diana, who personified the Hunter; Vulcan, the Craftsman; and Mars, the Warrior.

years Joan had felt physically unwell and was angry at God because she felt she didn't deserve her illness. Basically, she consulted me because she wanted proof that God was mistaken. She hadn't done anything wrong. It was other people. Why was God punishing her?

"I noticed that you had several abortions in your twenties," I said, as a prelude to talking about Joan's lack of forgiveness for herself.

"Well, it wasn't my fault I got pregnant!" she interrupted.

I realized in that moment that Joan was living out a very damaging kind of Victim **archetype**. It drastically needed changing. Trying to reason with a fully engaged Victim is like trying to reason with someone under the influence of drugs or alcohol. It's a waste of good breath.

During a reading I see the predominant archetype that you are living from. It could be the Victim, Knight, Scholar, Peacemaker, Princess, Judge, Rebel, Mystic, Artist, Earth Mother, Goddess, Hermit, Saboteur, Healer, or Slave. An archetype is shorthand for the way in which someone is predisposed to act and react in the world. For example, someone with a low vibration of the Princess archetype wants everything done for her and given to her without having to lift a finger. A low vibration of the Knight archetype is found in a man who thinks it's up to him to save damsels in distress: He is attracted to women with huge problems so he can rush in and solve them.

Sometimes there are two or three archetypes competing for the top slot. Joan's chief archetype was the Victim, but her Wounded Child archetype was struggling to be seen, heard, and pitied. I decided to find out where her Wounded Child came from.

I scanned Joan's past and saw that her brothers generally ignored her and wouldn't play with her. Her father and mother were busy with their own agendas and had little time for Joan either. She had many "I don't feel well" days as a child, which brought her some measure of attention from her parents, but overall she felt very lost, alone, and unloved. Joan had created (as many do) God in the image of her dominant parent: Dad. Apparently, God had no time for her either, because her prayers asking for a friend went unanswered. Because of Joan's archetypal makeup, she felt victimized and ignored by God. She concluded that God took care of everyone but her. And that clearly was not her fault!

When Joan grew up, she still blamed God for her woes. Her prayers were asked and answered by her Victim archetype, and they went like this: "God, why won't you make me feel better?" Answer: "Because you're too busy with others." But Joan would take no responsibility for her situation and concluded that God was ignoring her.

"See," she whined, "God has no time for me and doesn't even answer my prayers." Joan was so trapped in her beliefs and unwilling to change them, she couldn't have heard God if he shouted with a megaphone from a burning bush. Because of her attachment to being a helpless victim, she was more concerned with playing the injured party and complaining about being victimized than being open to help.

Even worse, Joan was so attached to being a victim, she couldn't entertain the possibility that she could be spiritually responsible and change her life. Her Victim archetype just wanted to keep blaming God for her physical condition. In addition, Joan enjoyed being unwell: She loved the attention and the chaos inherent in all those office visits and hospital tests. She wasn't about to give up such a rewarding pursuit.

Complaining gave Joan the attention she craved, but her satisfaction was fleeting. Her "poor me" act eventually wore thin, and people – including her family – distanced themselves from her. Hurt and frustrated, she screamed at God one day, "This is all your fault!" And she never spoke to God again. Her crown chakra shut down. Her life force dwindled. She was caught between death and life.

Too "ill" to do anything but still hell-bent on blaming others for her woes, Joan looked miserable and felt miserable. My scan of her energy system revealed no physical illness, but she was indeed sick – spiritually sick.

Sadly, Joan had no desire to do anything about it. She didn't want to get well. It was more important to her to rail at God and to be right. Joan is a classic example of what I call the "overrule" phenomenon. A client's soul always overrules a healer's. A laying on of hands would have had the same effect on Joan as swinging a rubber chicken over her head. Nothing would heal this woman because she did not want to be healed. She wanted validation that she was right and she wanted vengeance against God. Joan wore her victimhood like a badge of honor, reveling in her misery and avenging herself by proclaiming God's inadequacy and his indifference to her.

This is an example of what happens when you turn away from God and into yourself. You – your pain, suffering, beliefs, and woes – become more important than your relationship with the source of all life and unconditional love. Joan reasoned this way: God didn't love her enough to keep her well. That was why she had gotten sick. And that was that. She wasn't willing to work on getting well, she wasn't willing to look at her tribal beliefs about God, and she certainly wasn't willing to work on having a relationship with God.

I told Joan that I saw no physical illness in her body, but I had seen an energetic illness.

"Well, what is it?" she snapped, clearly annoyed that I had

turned out to be as "stupid" as all her other medical consultants. "It is more important for you to be right than to be well. You thoroughly enjoy being a victim, and you are not willing to be spiritually responsible for your life."

Needless to say, Joan thought it was my fault that she had gotten such a "bad" reading.

◆ ◆ ◆

Earlier in this chapter, I mentioned **energetic suicide**. I see this disorder more than I care to admit. In energetic suicide, there is no energy moving through the chakras. It often begins as a complete blockage in the first, second, or third chakras, which then progresses to a complete blockage in all three. Or it can start with the seventh, or crown, chakra. Once your crown chakra is closed, all the rest of your chakras begin to shut down, causing emotional and spiritual death, which can eventually lead to physical death.

The symptoms of energetic suicide include fatigue, mild depression, hopelessness, aimlessness, a sense of futility, and feeling trapped. This may be well disguised. Clients with energetic suicide have walked into my office smiling, joking, and talking about their wonderful futures and their next big adventures. Despite their words, I can't pick up the vibration of excitement in their energetic blueprint. Instead what I see is an energetic listlessness and a person trying desperately to feel alive. Often, these are quite busy people who seem to be doing a lot, but who in reality are merely walking through

Energetic Suicide

Choosing to cut yourself off from your soul, your guidance, and God. The result is that no energy flows through your chakras. You feel empty, useless, and exhausted. You go through the motions of life without any passion.

the motions of their daily lives.

Jessica, a psychologist in her late sixties, came for a session hoping I could psychically identify her true passion. After hearing my diagnosis of energetic suicide, she tenaciously clung to and defended her delusions of happiness and a full life, claiming she was an extremely vibrant person. Jessica insisted that she found great meaning in her work and her grandchildren, and was only puzzled about why she hadn't found her true passion yet.

What I saw instead was that Jessica was waiting to feel alive, hoping that some external event would bring excitement to her life.

As she sat before me, Jessica's vibration was so low, I could barely detect it, but she flatly refused to entertain the possibility that her energetic blueprint did not match her description of herself. Living in this delusion prevented her from healing her energetic suicide and finding her passion. Denial, as they say, is not just a river in Egypt — it can be a deadly foe.

People with energetic suicide are literally emotionally dead

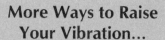

More Ways to Raise Your Vibration...

- Sing.
- Pray.
- Ask for and listen to divine guidance.
- Give thanks for the blessings you have, and the gifts and talents you possess.
- Laugh.
- Light candles.
- Love a pet.
- Be emotionally intimate and present with another.
- Give of yourself.

...or Lower It

- Deny that God exists.
- Never pray.
- Take your blessings for granted.
- Don't listen to your soul.
- Complain.
- Be a victim.
- Blame others.
- Seek vengeance.

and therefore incapable of true intimacy with another being. This added to Jessica's hidden feelings of loneliness and disconnection. Owning her energetic blueprint was essential to begin healing and ultimately find her passion.

Other clients with energetic suicide come in with a vague sense that something is not quite right. They might admit to feeling somewhat lost or mildly depressed. They acknowledge that something seems to be missing from their lives and life feels somewhat flat, even though they've done everything right and attained their goals. Even with this insight, when I ask them to tell me honestly what percentage of them, from zero to one hundred, wants to be here on the earth, they are often surprised at the low number they give.

What causes energetic suicide? Writing God or your Higher Power out of your life, losing a loved one or watching a good friend die, feeling like your life has lost all meaning, or ignoring the needs of your soul for a prolonged period of time. Each of these can shut down your chakra system.

A closed or partially closed crown chakra can result from ignoring or shutting God out of your life. When your crown chakra closes, you rarely receive inspiration and certainly have trouble hearing guidance. You become separate from a universal connection: love. I often find that people with energetic suicide are constantly searching for something, trying new workshops or ideas or spiritual philosophies, but always moving on to the next promise of fulfillment. Their souls are restless because they are separated from God, so they wander in search of something – anything – to fill that deep longing for the love that we all crave.

Sometimes that longing becomes a terrible ache when a mate, a good friend, or a loved one is dying. In this vulnerable state, people often rail against God and deny themselves a true sense of comfort. I treated a woman who energetically linked with her dying brother to hold on to the last morsels of love and connection. The pain of being alone was so great that she lost her magnetics for life. When a loved one dies, the ache can become a relentless wound without God's comfort, and a piece of you goes with the person – you've heard of people dying of a broken heart. You become deadened and simply wait for your own death. When I treat people like this, it is essential to help them call back and reclaim that lost part of themselves so they can live.

Dying can also be metaphoric. The age-old questions "What is the meaning of my life" or "Why am I here?" plague many people. Feeling adrift without any purpose is the beginning of energetic shutdown. It can feel like your life is over. Many people don't know what to do with their lives, mainly because they can't or won't listen to guidance. Usually this is because their guidance flies in the face of their cherished tribal beliefs. They would rather be one of the walking dead than step away from the tribe or ask God back into their lives.

Being separate from God is like living in your ego. In other words, it's fighting against your soul. Your soul is your connection to God, while your ego is your connection to your own wants and needs. When you ignore your soul, you are fighting against your highest good, which puts you in constant conflict, drains your energy, and shuts down the chakra system. Call the soul your higher self, your inner wisdom, or whatever you want, it's all the same thing. I call it the smart part of us. When you don't listen to your soul, you are going against your true nature and you start to die.

Interestingly, people can exist in a mild state of energetic suicide for a long time. They may not be physically ill. Even so, energetic suicide is a serious condition and is more urgent to treat than an actual physical illness. First you lose the richness of life and begin an existence without passion or joy. Eventually you lose the will to live, a condition that can be more damaging and life-threatening than cancer. In the early stages of energetic suicide, many people have vague symptoms but no definitive illness. People can live with varying degrees of energetic suicide for a number of years, but eventually the complete shutdown of their chakra energy system will result in disease or death.

The first step in treating energetic suicide is determining what percentage of you really wants to live. (Being in denial prevents you from healing.) You can't want to live for your mate, your parents, or your children. It is the percentage of you that wants to be here *for you* that determines whether you will heal. Once you are aware that you are experiencing energetic suicide, everything changes – you can recognize that adrift feeling, the lack of passion, the vague uncaring about a life with seemingly no meaning. You know that this is actually energetic suicide and it is treatable. You no longer feel trapped, resigned, or doomed.

Knowing what percentage of you wants to live opens you up to choices and is extremely empowering – it causes something to shift inside you. This knowledge allows you to make a choice about dying or living a life based on guidance and flow, replete with passion and joy. If a person decides on life, my next priority is opening her chakra system and simultaneously reconnecting her with God by praying with her. Having her do daily rituals to raise her vibration (such as praying gratitude) continues the healing process.

The key to recovery is identifying that one is suffering from energetic suicide. This allows the person to consciously choose to live, take responsibility for her life, and follow the necessary steps to reclaim it.

CHAPTER 14

Living Guidance

*A life without guidance is like a life without sight, hearing,
and smell, without wonderful dinners, sunsets, or
music, without laughter, without song, without joy.*

Question: When is guidance not guidance?
Answer: When it doesn't come from God but rather from your own head or ego.

Question: How does one know if it is guidance or our ego speaking?

Answer: Guidance is clear, short, and sweet. The ego engages in a lot of chatter, discussion, and rationalizing; it is very noisy and chaotic.

Question: Why would anyone doubt or not follow guidance?

Answer: Because he doesn't like what he's hearing!

During my trip to Peru, I had a hard time listening to my guidance. I kept doubting that the guidance coming to me really *was* divine guidance because I didn't want to listen to it. Even after returning to California – healthy, strong, and completely cured of multiple sclerosis – I struggled with how to live the guidance I was given. I knew God wanted me to use my gifts full-time, but I had no clue where to begin. Get a 900 number? Put an ad in the paper? Hang out a shingle? I began to worry: *I don't know the first thing about making a living as a Medical Intuitive. What if nobody comes? How will I pay my bills?*

Herein lay my first mistake: I was making assumptions about my guidance. I assumed that all the details of my new life would be clearly set out – even the steps would be outlined for me. However, you cannot follow divine guidance by thinking in physical terms. Guidance is a path to follow; all you are supposed to do is start walking. The details become clearer the farther you walk. My second mistake was to falter in my trust of my guidance –and hence of God. I kept panicking, thinking *I need to pay the rent and eat! How will I do that?* But again, I was thinking in physical terms, not divine terms. When I felt afraid, I railed aloud at my angels, "If you want me to follow my guidance, tell me what steps to take!"

Their response was always the same: *Simply trust.*

Yeah, what do they know? I thought. *They don't eat and they don't need to pay rent. They may think this is funny, but I don't!*

When I considered the guidance I had been given, I vacillated between fear and awe, but I always came back to that moment at the rock in Peru when I had given my word. The sign I had demanded from God had indubitably come, and, darn it, I was going to keep my word despite my fear. This is also known as courage – choosing to make something else (in this case, the integrity of giving my word) more important than one's fear. Once I gained that courage, I became open to all possibilities and opportunities – a stance that finally enabled God to present me with what I needed for my journey, which I'll tell you about in a moment. The lesson I learned was that I had to make something else (in this case, following my guidance) more important than my fear.

A few weeks after getting back from Peru, I was walking on the beach with my friend Carol, a sparkler of a woman. Carol had the absolute charisma to make people feel special and loved. Her sense of humor was infectious. The two of us were inseparable and incorrigible, the Lucy and Ethel of 1990s Southern California. I liked to think I was Ethel, the one who was always getting coaxed into hot water by her screwball friend, but in truth Carol and I shared the role of Lucy.

As we walked, I picked up the energetic signature of cancer in Carol's energy field. I gently told her what I perceived. She immediately made an appointment with her doctor. Two doctors told her she was fine, but the third doctor found cancer. By the time Carol had gotten in to see him, the cancer had entered her body.* She was diagnosed with breast cancer. Carol made the decision to combine Western and complementary medicine, and started chemotherapy soon afterwards.

One morning I accompanied Carol to the chemotherapy treatment room while an IV dripped toxic chemicals into her bloodstream. Next to Carol another woman was also receiving chemo. When I looked over at her, I inadvertently read her en-

---

* From the time I pick up the signs of illness in your energy field, it can take anywhere from three days to three months to actually enter your body. For example, I once did a reading for a psychotherapist on the East Coast. Based on what I saw in her energy field, I told her to make a choice right now about retiring. She was in conflict with her soul, which was frantic for her to get out of a job that consistently drained and angered her. I saw she had about four days before she would get leukemia. She made the decision that she would continue working for a few more years. A week later she was diagnosed with leukemia.

ergy field. Normally I would never have let this happen. I learned early on to be scrupulous about never reading anyone without her express permission. But I was distracted by my concern about Carol, and the information came to me before I realized what was happening.

This woman's friend was sitting at the table next to me. I leaned over and asked her gently, "Is your friend in there estranged from her mother?"

A frown creased the woman's forehead, then was quickly replaced by a look of complete surprise. "You *couldn't* know that about her!" she exclaimed. "You've never met her... but you're right."

The woman getting chemo was named Lindsey, and what I saw in her energy field was an emotional tug of war. Lindsey secretly hated her mother because she thought she treated her like a helpless child and did not recognize her potential or her achievements. Lindsey even secretly fantasized once about her mother having a stroke and being left helpless. Rather than accept and resolve her anger at her mother, she felt she was evil for having had such thoughts. She also had a deep need to be part of the family again. The inner conflict between Lindsay's longing and her hatred, along with her refusal to forgive her mother, had lowered her vibration until it had resonated with the vibration of cancer.

Still a little distracted, I told her friend, Marie, that I was a Medical Intuitive, and I could read and interpret people's energy.

"What would help Lindsey heal?" Marie asked urgently.

"First, she needs to call her mother so they can start talking. Tell her to find a way to forgive her mother and get her secret out."

"What secret?" Marie asked.

"Just tell her what I said," I replied. "She'll know."

"Alright," Marie said decisively. "And I'll make sure she listens!"

To make a long story short, Lindsey made peace with her mother, rejoined the family, and is happier than she's ever been. She completed her course of chemotherapy. The cancer is gone from her body. She's not in remission; she's cured.[*]

◆   ◆   ◆

As it turned out, Lindsey needed me in order to move ahead with her life journey, and I needed Lindsey's friend Marie in order to move ahead with mine. Marie worked for a very well-known and respected acupuncturist. She was also a born networker and seemed to know about three-quarters of the population of Southern California. Thanks to her, I soon could not fit into my schedule all the people who were calling me for readings. Not long after, people in other states had heard of me. I started traveling and teaching. I even did readings by telephone for people in other countries.

That's the power of guidance. I hadn't had to write a business plan or put ads in the newspaper. Although I had started out ignoring my guidance and ending up with MS, once I chose to follow my guidance and stopped fighting God, I had a spontaneous healing and met a woman who would be instrumental in helping me accept my calling to be a full-time Medical Intuitive. What's more, my connection with this woman began because I

---

[*] This is a good place to point out that I do not disdain Western medicine. I think people should use whatever helps them heal. My friend Carol, for example, got some benefit from her chemotherapy. She also got tremendous healing from our work together. In two different hands-on sessions with me, she experienced spontaneous healing, only to have her cancer return each time because she chose not to change the tribal beliefs that were lowering her vibration and opening her chakras to illness. Staying loyal to her family's values was more important to her than living a long life.

was doing something kind – without any expectation of a pay-back – for a sick friend. That's how God works.

This experience taught me that you have to trust your guid-ance no matter how scared you are. Guidance is divine and it may not make sense in terms of the physical world. You have to follow it anyway. Don't worry. *I guarantee that if you listen to your guidance, you will always end up at least ten times happier than you were before.*

Your guidance is always trying to get your attention. In fact, you have to work quite diligently if you want to keep your dis-tance from your Higher Power. You must work even harder to ignore the many signs put before you to aid your spiritual growth.

While it is true that God will not interfere or swoop down to save the day, God will readily participate in your life. God *wants* to have a relationship with you. This begins the moment you ask for help and open your heart. Having an open heart en-ables you to hear the guidance you so desperately need.

Having a relationship with God works the same way that healing does. If you don't want to be healed, there is not a healer on this planet who can override your free will. Similarly, if you choose to block out God, your choice will not be overridden by divine intervention. You must choose to have a relationship with God just as you must choose to heal. That is the essence of free will, and it is what separates us from animals. We have choices. Our lives are not based simply upon instinct and survival.

Our Higher Power is always available to us. We simply need to reach out and ask for help. Unfortunately, for some people it's not that "simple." They pray for help yet lack sincerity. Take it from my personal experience, if your prayers aren't sincere, you won't get a clear answer.

For example, during that period of my life when my health

first declined, I prayed to know what was wrong with me and what I needed to do to get better. Two or three months passed but I could hear no guidance. I was frustrated and confused, as I had never before prayed for guidance without getting an answer. So I took a long hard look at myself and my prayers, and I realized that if I were completely honest with myself, I didn't really want to know what was wrong with me. I was afraid to find out. So even though I was praying for an answer, a small part of me was whispering, "If it's serious, I don't want to know."

When I realized what I was doing, I made a conscious choice to learn the truth about my health, and I prayed with honesty and sincerity to discover what my diagnosis was. From that moment, the world opened up for me. Medical tests that had been scheduled months down the road suddenly became available the next day due to a cancellation. I received my answer within the week.

The key is that when you pray, you have to mean it. Don't ask for guidance if you already have your mind made up (as I did when I was a nurse who wouldn't give up nursing), or if you only want guidance that fits into your present life (ditto). You will always get a response if you simply ask. But the answer will not always be one that you are happy with. Don't ask to be molded by God unless you are ready to make the changes necessary to decrease your separation from God.

Sometimes those changes relate to your tribe, which consists of the family you grew up with, the family you have created around you now, such as mates and friends, and the family of all of us here on the planet. There is an unwritten law on which all tribes are based: Follow our rules and all is well. Break them and you will be rejected, orphaned, even stoned. So you stick with the "safety" of the tribe. You follow its rules and believe its beliefs. Unfortunately, when you stick with the tribe, you are stuck with their level of spiritual evolution, too. All tribe members evolve spiritually at the same rate, be it fast or sluggishly slow.

Let me give you an example. Briana's tribe believed if you worked hard, you would never fail. If you did fail, it was never due to external factors, it was because *you* hadn't worked hard enough. Briana, being human, did fail at things sometimes. Normally, this would have been okay: making mistakes is how we learn. But her tribe's belief condemned her for her failures. And she condemned herself. This put Briana in a perpetual no-win situation: She could never grab the brass ring. Her self-esteem was lower than low. Her confidence was nonexistent. No matter what went wrong, it was always her fault.

That brass ring was like a noose around Briana's neck. Remember, you magnetize events and people based upon your beliefs and the clutter in your energy field. This clutter can include comments from others that have lowered your self-esteem (like "You're a failure" or "You're nobody") or not forgiving yourself for a time when you used poor judgment. This clutter will help you magnetize people who will treat you like dirt (thus "proving" that you're worthless) and are judgmental toward you for (supposedly) being stupid, lacking integrity, whatever.

Because Briana had low self-esteem (due to clutter in her energy field), she magnetized people who were in impossible situations. When Briana would try to help them, she would fail. For example, she tried for years to make her husband happy, yet he was quite content with his Martyr and Victim archetypes. From Briana's point of view, his misery was another one of her failures.

She even magnetized a healing profession where cure is a rare word: psychology. As I said earlier, no one can be healed unless she wants to be. Imagine going into a profession (as Briana did) where people claim they want to feel better, but in truth do not. Your efforts to help these people would meet with only limited success. So, as hard as Briana worked and as much as she gave her patients, many of them continued to suffer. They had good days and bad days, but they never healed. The sight of their pain – which Briana saw as her failure to provide the right treatment – quietly reinforced for her the feeling that she was a failure.

Briana had unconsciously set up a no-win career situation for herself to give credence to the tribal belief that if she failed, it was because she hadn't worked hard enough. As a result, she worked harder and harder with her patients, and gave more and more of her time and energy – until she burned out. The tribal belief that working really, really hard is the road to success turned Briana into a hamster running on a wheel. No matter how fast she ran, she never got anywhere.

But that hamster wasn't alone in her cage. Her family was with her. By adhering to their tribal belief, Briana would remain a welcome member of the tribe. She would evolve at their rate – and work long and hard without getting the brass ring. Letting go of her family's tribal belief would get her evicted from the cage, but it would spur her spiritual growth. That was because the tribal belief was keeping Briana separate from God. The belief was all about ego and pride and hard work. Ego says, *I must work harder or I am a failure.* Pride says, *I can't fail.* Listening to guidance means quieting the ego and giving yourself to service for God. It says, *What do you want me to do today?* (And it might not include hard work and sacrifice.)

God didn't write those tribal rules or ask Briana to be true to them. She chose to adhere to them so she would win her tribe's approval.

When I met Briana and learned about her situation, I asked her a question I often find myself asking my clients: "Are you willing to entertain the idea that your tribe's belief is inhibiting or contrary to your spiritual growth?" Briana said yes, but I wasn't sure she had fully understood. We talked about it some more until it was clear she wanted to evolve spiritually no matter the cost. Briana took a hard look at her tribal belief that all failure is a result of not working hard enough and decided she didn't want to live like that anymore. Her attachment to her tribe had become less important than her attachment to God.

Did the tribe like it when Briana cut her work hours in half? Absolutely not! There was hell to pay. Her parents became terrified for her and responded with anger and criticism. Her husband became jealous and angry of her newfound freedom and lashed out at her. He felt he deserved to work less, too, but he wasn't willing to make choices that would bring him that freedom.

Why does the tribe react so strongly? Because if everyone were to disregard the contradictory and inhibiting beliefs of the tribe, it would cease to have power over others. A tribe cannot afford to have many freethinkers. If members of the tribe decide to shed the tribal beliefs and break away, the survival of the tribe is at risk. Tribes exist because there is strength – and safety – in numbers. Survival and safety are core needs for human beings, and we are used to getting these needs met by sticking with our tribes.

There's another way to achieve safety and ensure your survival: Give up the tribal beliefs that keep you separated from God.

When Briana decided to make her relationship with God more important than her fear of being rejected by her tribe, she was basically making the same decision I did when I returned to California from Peru. (In my case, I decided to make following my guidance more important than my fear of not being able to pay my bills.) Although bucking your tribe's laws is scary, there comes a point when you must decide which tribal laws and traditions feed your soul and give you life-enhancing energy, and which don't. You are not meant to live at a low vibration. Your guidance and connection with God will raise your vibration, if only you will listen. You must look at your unconscious behavior and the choices you've made that are based upon the tribal way, and decide if they are good for you or not. Do you want to evolve spiritually and be closer to God, or do you want to remain safely ensconced within the tribe and keep your distance from God? Ironically, many tribes with a stated spiritual purpose have tribal beliefs and laws that actually keep people separate from God. For example, *you must use a priest to receive absolution from God; suffering is noble; God's love for you is dependent upon your actions; there's only one true religion or path to God.*

While stepping away from the tribe is never easy, stepping toward God is always rewarding. The tribe will not embrace or cheer you on, but the angels will. I see too many people who wait until their parents have passed on to take the plunge and explore their own beliefs. When they do, they begin to live for the first time – but they are already in their late fifties or sixties. They may not have the energy to fully enjoy their newfound freedom. Or they may already be battling a debilitating or life-threatening illness.

I hope you don't decide to wait that long. A healthy, joyful, and satisfying life is available *now*. Guidance is available *now*. God is ready to bestow grace upon us *now*.

Just open your heart and ask for it. Your life as you know it *can* be different.

CHAPTER 15

Is a Reading Right for You?

There are a number of common questions and concerns that I hear from people who are considering a reading with me. I want to devote this chapter to answering them, because you may have these questions and concerns too, whether you are considering working with me or another Medical Intuitive. One note before I begin: Most Medical Intuitives are not also spiritual healers. I am. This means that I work differently than other Medical Intuitives. So when the answers I give are specifically about my practice rather than medical intuition in general, I will make that clear.

What can a reading do for me?

A reading by a reputable Medical Intuitive can identify any physical illness already in your body. We can also see illness in your energy system before it manifests in your physical body, which Western medicine cannot yet do. Early detection via medical intuition allows you to point your physician in the right direction for diagnosis and treatment, even if all the clinical indicators show there is nothing wrong with you. In addition, you can begin working with the emotional origins and patterns linked to your illness long before a Western diagnosis is available.

When working with the emotional components of illness, I look into your past and help you understand the incidents or trauma from childhood that set the stage for your situation. I can see the decisions you made, the perceptions you developed about yourself, and what you need to do to move on. People who have blank spots in their memories from childhood often get a feeling of validation and wholeness from knowing the facts about their past.

When you are facing not a physical illness, but a lack of joy or success in some area of your life, I can tell you what's in your way. This is an important aspect of my own work and I call it identifying your shadow. When you understand the unconscious patterns of behavior that lower your vibration and prevent you from achieving your dreams, you can decide whether to continue in those patterns or not. This kind of reading is hugely empowering. It brings to light the unconscious factors that are driving you, and you learn exactly what choices you need to make to improve your life.

If I am doing a healing with you as well as a reading, I raise your vibrational frequency, which, if accepted and embraced, often leads to a spontaneous healing of your physical, emotional, or spiritual illness.

Why would I schedule a reading?

There are several reasons for scheduling a reading with a Medical Intuitive:

◆ Your physician can't seem to figure out why you've lost your pep or verve for life.

♦ You have an intuitive sense that something is wrong with your body and you want to heal it.

♦ You're stuck or bored and find yourself just going through the motions of living. You wish your life were different, but don't know what to do.

♦ You'd like to know why you still do the unhealthy things you do, despite your best intentions to do things differently.

♦ You are looking for a deeper connection with your Higher Power and with yourself.

♦ You want something more in your life, or are looking for success in a particular area or endeavor.

♦ You are looking for a relationship or want answers about the relationship you are in.

♦ You know you are missing something and long for someone to be honest with you about what it is.

♦ Your life is great, and you want to make sure it stays that way!

♦ Your intuition is telling you it's the right thing to do.

What kinds of people come for a reading?

All kinds. People from every socioeconomic level and widely different careers. People with graduate degrees and people still in high school. People who believe in a sixth sense and people who don't. Business people who are looking for ways to increase their success, women who can't seem to get pregnant, people of all ages looking to be healthy or find out why they seem to be stuck in life.

Generally, the factor that unites all of the people who come to me for a reading is this: They have already sought help from doctors, coaches, therapists, and/or spiritual teachers in the traditional or Western realm for their medical, emotional, psychological, practical, and/or spiritual problems, but have gotten limited or no results. After all the searching and money they've spent, they have nothing to show for it. They are at the end of their rope and can't stand it anymore.

How do I know if a reading is right for _me_?

Since I do not give you _my_ opinion on what's wrong but merely report what your body and energy system are telling me, my work goes to the heart of your issues very quickly. Your core objections to healing are compassionately exposed. This can be unsettling. So even though my style is gentle and loving, you need to schedule your first appointment with me for when you feel courageous enough to laser down to the very bottom of what blocks you from healing.

If you're uncertain about whether you are ready to heal quickly, or if slow and gradual is the best way for you to work on your issues, then I recommend doing prep work with a good psychotherapist before getting a reading with me.

Are there people who shouldn't get a reading?

Any form of healing, whether it be physical, emotional, or spiritual, requires commitment, compliance with the healer's instructions, and the desire to heal. Learning about your energetic blueprint is invaluable if you want to change your life for the better or achieve your goals. If you want to get a reading just because seeing a clairvoyant is an interesting way to get information about yourself, that's great. But if you don't plan on doing anything with that information, consult another Medical Intuitive. I am interested only in working with people who want to physically, emotionally, or spiritually heal and are willing to make changes that will improve their lives.

What happens in a reading?

When I read your energy, it's simple and direct. I sit across from you, and while talking to you I scan your physical body for illness, past surgeries, or pain. I also read your emotional body, your spiritual body, and, most importantly, your energy field. I do not need to be physically present with a client; I only need his permission.

During a reading I receive a tremendous amount of information in a matter of two to three minutes. Generally, I see a running video of significant events from childhood, and I identify the predominant (and often negative) belief you carry about yourself, which affects all arenas of your life, such as career, relationships, and financial affairs. I also see your dominant archetypes and the unconscious traumas, decisions, and emotional patterns contributing to your physical, emotional, and/or spiritual illness. In addition, I identify for you the one priority task that will reverse these patterns.

What is your personal goal in reading someone?

I want to make you aware of your unconscious choices so you are free to make new choices that will bring you in alignment with your soul. Making such choices is the beginning of spiritual responsibility, and aligning with your soul is one of the most powerful, liberating, and healing experiences you will ever have — it connects you to your Higher Power.

You see, when I read your energy, I see who you are and I see the person you are meant to be. This shows me the ways in which your energy is not matching up. It's like seeing two pictures overlaying each other. The main picture – who you are meant to be – is clear and bright. It shows your highest expression, your most exciting possibilities. The other is the energy you are expressing now, which usually ranges from muddy to dark. I want to help you understand the muddiness so that you can change it. My goal is to see you become the person you are meant to be, the one who is clear, bright, and filled with God's love.

How do I find a reputable Medical Intuitive?

Referral, referral, and referral. You wouldn't pick a cardiologist out of the phone book, so why would you call a psychic hotline? Talk to people who know the Medical Intuitive. Make sure she is affiliated with the local community, perhaps with physicians and psychologists. If a doctor or psychologist is referring you, it means there is a working health-care-team relationship.

Good Medical Intuitives rarely do psychic fairs and don't advertise in the back of the *National Enquirer*. Check their qualifications, background, and training. Having no connection to medicine is a definite deal breaker!

My years as a registered nurse in the field of emergency trauma were critical in shaping my own practice. It is essential for a Medical Intuitive to understand anatomy and physiology, and some microbiology wouldn't hurt. If you've never seen a cancer cell under a microscope, how would you know what you were seeing when it showed up in your scan?

How can I tell if a Medical Intuitive is any good?

There are six telltale signs of a poor practitioner:

1. **Asking too many questions.** Recently I decided to experience a reading by another Medical Intuitive to see what was happening in my professional world. I con-

tacted a fairly well-known intuitive and was sent a thir-
teen-page questionnaire to answer before the reading.
After perusing the questions, I found myself wondering
why a *clairvoyant* would need me to tell them things
about myself. When a Medical Intuitive asks you a lot of
questions, it's not a good sign.

2. **Asking for more money during a session.** When a
    Medical Intuitive asks you for an additional fee to con-
    tinue giving you information during a session – especially
    when you are just getting to the important part of the
    reading – head for the door.

3. **Coming from darkness.** If the person you are consult-
    ing is connected to anything dark or evil, run. You can
    recognize someone like this because his ego enters the
    room before he does. Such people are very concerned
    with looking important and mystical and powerful. And
    they don't need to wear a headdress to pull that off.

4. **Having no medical background.** If a person claims to
    be a Medical Intuitive, please check out her medical
    background. Many so-called Medical Intuitives don't
    know on which side of the body the liver is found be-
    cause they've never taken anatomy or physiology, seen a
    liver, or had any medical experience.

5. **Lack of compassion.** Intuitive information is not some-
    thing one blurts out simply because it is there. I am sad-
    dened by the display of some Medical Intuitives almost
    flippantly calling out diagnoses such as depression. My
    first question to that intuitive would be, is it a clinical
    depression? Have you looked at the state of the person's
    serotonin receptors? Alternatively, is it spiritual depres-
    sion? The treatment modalities are quite different and

specific for each diagnosis. Or, when the vibration for cancer is identified, it is not enough to simply say, "You have cancer." It is important for the Medical Intuitive to know if there is metastasis or if the cancer is encapsulated and contained. If a client is considering surgery, this information is highly relevant. I have also heard intuitives blurt out information regarding childhood abuse they have picked up on during a reading. I think this is as unethical as doing a reading without consent. What if the client does not have a good support system? What if he is not working with a therapist? What if she is financially dependent on her past abuser? The gift of medical intuition carries with it moral responsibility. It is not a party game.

6. **Lack of commitment to the profession.** I hate to say this, since I was once in this position myself, but when a person is doing this kind of work part-time, it speaks volumes. You don't want to receive a reading from someone who does it as a hobby or because he thinks he has some intuitive gifts but hasn't bothered to hone them by doing intensive training, such as interning with a Medical Intuitive, doing readings every day to learn about the limits of his intuition and learn what the different frequencies of vibrations mean, and verifying his readings with test results from Western medicine. When you work with an amateur, you are going to get exactly what you pay for.

If chakras get sick before the body, why doesn't my doctor worry about them?

It takes a special talent to read the chakras, and your doctor probably doesn't have it. In addition, the mind-body-spirit connection, while not new, has yet to fully catch on in some areas of medicine. Western physicians are true scientists – they want studies and numbers before they accept a new paradigm like energy medicine.

Other frequently asked questions

Do you go into a trance during a reading? Nope. My eyes don't roll up in the back of my head, my voice doesn't change, and I don't channel people from the past. I am very present with you.

Will my secrets be revealed? Yes, because they are part of your energetic profile. I will see if you are gay, had an abortion, have experienced sexual, physical, or emotional abuse, are having an affair, or are embezzling from your company. Since all energy is neutral, I don't judge your actions, belief, or ideas. I simply report to you what I see and what effect it is having on your energy system. Secrets severely drain your system.

After the reading, then what? I give you step-by-step instructions on where and how to begin your transformative and healing journey.

Do I come back for another reading? That depends. Some people need only one reading, others need many. No matter which is true for you, you will receive a clear and concise map showing the steps needed to reach your goals. I always say to trust your intuition: You'll know if you need to come back.

Can you tell if my new business will succeed or help me make more money? Yes. I can tell you what stands between your desires and your ability to make them happen.

Do you read children? Yes. I do a reading with the child and his mother and then speak directly to the mom. However, I always get psychic permission from the child the day before the reading.

Are you always reading people on the street? No, I've learned to shut down my gift. I find it unethical to read a person without consent. However, because I perceive cancer by its smell, it's the one skill I can't shut down.

How can you see the past, when it has already happened? For me, time is not linear. It is a spiral. The past, present, and future are occurring at the same time. I'm not actually looking forward or backward. I'm just looking.

Can you tell when someone is going to die? When the death is inevitable, yes. When a person has choices to avoid it, no.

Can you tell if I'm going to win the lottery? When appropriate, I look three to five years into the future, but generally my focus is on the present. This is where we live and this is where we make choices to improve our life, health, and relationships. I decided long ago to use my gifts to heal and to teach. I prefer helping people to align with their souls, allowing them to find their true calling. If all you want is your future foretold, it shows me you are not interested in taking spiritual responsibility for your life or being empowered to make new choices. It screams of wanting a "quick fix" for your life. What I offer you is the best fix for your life: An understanding of who you are, why you do what you do, and how you can easily change it if you want.

Do you work with people in psychotherapy? Yes, my work can be a complement to almost any kind of psychotherapy. My readings offer tremendous insight to the therapist, who can then help her client make changes.

Can a reading make me well? In more ways than one. You can heal emotionally, spiritually, or physically by owning the ways you are lowering your vibration and choosing to change it.

Is it true you are a healer? Yes, in the broadest sense, though I usually prefer to be called a teacher. I heal through guidance – it is God who is actually doing the healing, I am merely the conduit. The overall mechanism of healing is something I call LUMOS.* Using LUMOS™, I teach you how to heal the chakras, thus raising your vibration. When you have learned to raise your vibration, trust your Higher Power, and let go of old, limiting beliefs, your healing is underway.

I've heard you can do spontaneous healing of illness. Is this true? Yes, there have been many spontaneous healings, but certain conditions apply: You have to want healing and your energy must be focused in the present, not the past. You can't be beating yourself up for what happened in the past. You can't be reliving traumas from the past. You must be fully present and in your body. You can't be worrying too much about the future either or your energy goes there. People who live in their heads are not in their hearts. Nor are people who live in the past or the future. They are not present and open to receiving healing because they are too distracted.

In addition, all energy drains (such as having conflicts with your soul, carrying tribal beliefs that are not good for you, manipulating others from your second chakra, staying in abusive relationships, or staying in situations for which you have no magnetics) must be stopped. If not, any apparent healing you experience will just be a remission, not a true healing.

If I am supposed to facilitate a spontaneous healing, I am "told" in the moment and enable the healing through my connection with God. This raises the person's overall vibration so it no longer resonates with her illness. For a physical illness, a hands-on approach is usually necessary. For emotional and spiritual

---

* This term is explained on Page 128.

healing, it is not. I also teach people how to raise their own vibration, thus beginning the process.

**Do you have to believe in spontaneous healing to
have one?** No. Nor do you have to believe in God for God to
exist. But an open mind will surely speed up a healing.

**Can you heal me if I'm not in the same room with
you?** I do remote readings by phone for people around the
globe. I also do distance healing in the evening when a client is
sleeping or resting. Many people have healed an emotional issue
that has been plaguing them or had a spiritual crisis resolved via
my remote ministrations. Often people report they are aware of
my working on them.

**How can you know so much about me when I've told
you nothing?** This is part of my gift – the ability to see your entire energetic blueprint, which includes your past experiences,
your deepest thoughts about yourself, your fears, your gifts, and
your talents. All this information is in your chakras and your energy field.

Do you ever refuse to read a person? Yes. I believe that
doing a reading when someone wants one just for fun or has no
intention of using the information I provide is a waste of my
time. If I perceive this is the case, I will end the session almost
immediately. Also, I will not give the time of day to anyone who
is flirting with dark forces. Early on, the skeptics came to my office for proof of my abilities, and I obliged them. However, I
now have no desire to convince people my gifts are real. I'm only
interested in teaching you to experience the richest and healthiest
life possible.

Are you ever unable to read someone? Absolutely. A
person who says he wants to be read but is afraid may put up a
wall, and I will respect that. When people are wearing glasses, I
receive limited information about them, so I generally ask them

to take them off during the reading. Also, magnets and similar devices scatter electromagnetic energy, so I cannot pick up your energy signature easily when they are nearby. Last of all, when a person is very near death, she is so disconnected from her body that I receive very little information from her energy field, other than the fact that she is passing over. At that point, assisting her to leave her body becomes the priority, not getting information from her past.

Do I need to prepare for the reading? Just find a place that is quiet and away from magnets. Of course, having a sense of what you hope to accomplish with the reading can focus your energy and enhance the reading.

Are you a meditator or a vegetarian? Is that how you maintain your gift? No. I eat meat, adore dark chocolate, and don't meditate, but I do heartfelt prayer on a regular basis.

◆ ◆ ◆

A final note: I hope that after reading this book you can at least entertain the possibility that your life can be however you choose. Our choices do determine the nature of our lives. You can be happy and healthy or vengeful and unforgiving. It is all up to you.

Using the information from a Medical Intuitive's scan of your energetic blueprint in order to become spiritually responsible simply means being able to see new possibilities where once there were none. It means making choices that are good for you — letting go of limiting tribal beliefs, life-draining attitudes, and, yes, even unhealthy people and jobs.

This book is about changing your life for the better — easily, quickly, and for the most part effortlessly. As English philosopher James Allen so aptly wrote, "Circumstance does not the man make, but rather, man makes his circumstances. If you are not happy with your life, you can change it.

Christel Nani

Now Tell Me Your Success Stories!

There is nothing more uplifting and inspiring than hearing about a hero's journey.

We at the Center for Spiritual Responsibility want to share your story of healing with others. Tell us how you have used the principles of spiritual responsibility from either Nani's book or CDs to heal on the emotional, physical or spiritual level.

Perhaps you have let go of limiting tribal beliefs, transformed a damaging archetype, or healed an illness. Your story of courage and triumph will spread hope to others on the path of spiritual responsibility and healing.

Tell us how you have contributed to raising the vibration of the world by raising your vibration. Let us celebrate the successful journey of the hero within each of us.

I will share your stories with audiences, seminar participants, and in my future books and CDs.

Together, we can change our world for the better!

❖　❖　❖

When you write to us, please include a return address, e-mail or phone number where we can contact you if necessary.

Mail your stories to:

The Center for Spiritual Responsibility
132 N. El Camino Real, #412
Encinitas, CA 92024

Or email them to me: info@ChristelNani.com.

Glossary

Archetype

A predisposition to act and react in a certain way. For instance, when someone with a predominant Detective archetype encounters a child crying over a broken toy, she would ask, "How did that toy break?" Someone with a predominant Mother archetype would bend down and comfort the child. The gods and goddesses of ancient myths were personifications of archetypes. Some examples are Venus, who personified the Lover; Diana, who personified the Hunter; Vulcan, the Craftsman; and Mars, the Warrior.

Chakra

One of the seven major energy centers within the body. These energy centers are located near your spine and run from the top of your head (the "crown" chakra) to your tailbone (the "root" chakra). Each correlates to a major cluster of nerve cells (called ganglia) that branches out from your spinal cord. They also correlate to specific physical and emotional energies.

Crossing Over

When your soul leaves your physical body, usually at death, and goes to a place of pure love and pure spirit, which many call heaven.

Energetic Blueprint

Your energetic blueprint contains information about your beliefs, your perceptions about yourself and others, your connection with God, and your vibration. In short, it is a map that shows where you are putting your energy and whether those places are life-enhancing or not.

Energetic Signature

The unique electromagnetic vibration that emanates from each living thing. This vibration can be detected by certain people or by use of a spectroscopic microscope. The energetic signature serves as a unique identifier for every single being or substance that exists. Even identical twins have different energetic signatures.

Energetic Suicide

Choosing to cut yourself off from your soul, your guidance, and God. The result is that no energy flows through your chakras. You feel empty, useless, and exhausted. You go through the motions of life without any passion.

Energy Field

The area around the human body into which the electromagnetic energy that the cells of our bodies naturally produce is projected. The energy in this field vibrates at frequencies that change depending on your physical health and well-being. When you are healthy, the energy in this field vibrates at a high frequency. When you are unwell, it vibrates at a low frequency. Also called aura or etheric field.

Energy System

The human energy system has two parts: the electromagnetic energy field, which is located outside the body, and the seven major energy centers within the body, called chakras.

Flow

The state of serenity you feel when your heart, mind, and actions are in harmony with God's highest desire for you. People usually think of flow as a state when external things are going well. But flow is really about internal things going well. It's this internal state that smoothes the way for external success.

Guidance

Advice and instructions that come to you from God (or your Higher Power, the Divine, the Self, Spirit, or whatever term you are comfortable with). Your guidance will always point you in the direction of your greatest good because God is the source of the highest vibration of all: unconditional love.

Magnetics

Magnetics is a strong resonance for a specific situation. When you have magnetics for something, you feel vibrant and alive when you do it. Your vibration is high. You are acting in alignment with your soul's wishes. You can tell when you have magnetics for a relationship or a profession because you are energized by being in it.

When you lose magnetics for something, it exhausts you to do it. Your vibration drops. You are swimming upstream, ignoring your spiritual guidance. You can tell you have lost magnetics for a relationship or a profession because you feel drained by it.

Resonate

In the language of energy medicine, to resonate means to have energy that is vibrating at the same frequency as something else. It's like in a music store, when you pluck the G string on a guitar. Suddenly all the G strings on the other guitars begin to vibrate too. They are resonating with the frequency of the first string, responding to its vibration with an identical vibration of their own.

In very simple terms, this is how your body and psyche attract illness: When your vibration drops, whether for physical or emotional reasons, you resonate with the low vibration of illness.

Shadow

The buried and unconscious part of yourself that is running the show. It's what drives your behavior. It is the part that you have disavowed or disowned, perhaps because you are not aware of it. Uncovering what's in your shadow is crucial to your physical, emotional, and spiritual health because it can prevent you from healing. No matter what efforts you make to change your lifestyle or your beliefs, your true motives – which lie hidden in your shadow – will still be driving your behavior and will eventually sabotage all your good work.

Spiritual Responsibility

Taking responsibility for your life, no matter what illness, wounds, or problems you have and no matter who or what caused them. Being spiritually responsible is the polar opposite of identifying yourself as a victim.

Tribal Belief

An unconscious assumption instilled during childhood by your family, teachers, or religious training, such as *Girls aren't as smart as boys* or *Men owe it to their families to work hard and earn a lot of money*. Most tribal beliefs are energy-draining. Also, they don't feel like beliefs; to you, they are inescapable facts. Tribal beliefs reside in the root chakra, where they chip away at your sense of safety in the world and your desire to live.

Vibration

The frequency, ranging from high to low, of the electromagnetic energy that is emitted from all living cells.

Index

A

abuse, 70, 160
  child, 78, 127, 130
  domestic, 47, 49, 70
  sexual, 78, 112, 130
action, 60
adrenaline, 53
affirmations, 57, 58, 59, 64
afterlife, 9, 39, 42, 44
agnosticism, 127
allergies, 78
alternative medicine. *See*
  complementary medicine
anger, 50, 51, 53, 125, 144
appendicitis, 14, 46, 48, 52
archetype, 132, 157
  definition of, 167
  Detective, 132
  Knight, 133
  Martyr, 148
  Mother, 132
  Princess, 133
  Victim, 133–36, 148
  Wounded Child, 133
atheism, 127
aura. *See* energy field
awareness, 60

B

beliefs, 53, 54, 56, *See also*
  thoughts

effect on health, 55
high vibration, 54
linked to disease, 101–13
low vibration, 54
manifesting in your life, 60
negative, 69
power of, 55
predominant, 54, 58, 70, 80
predominant, cause of, 70
self-fulfilling, 54, 131
tribal. *See* tribal beliefs
unconscious, 60
blueprint, energetic. *See*
  energetic blueprint
boredom, 117, 118, 155

C

cancer, 1, 16, 21, 22, 31, 58, 61, 104, 143–45, 144, 160, 162
  breast, 103–7
  breast, as related to
    secrets, 104, 144
  breast, healing, 106
  breast, self-quiz, 106
  prostate, 75, 107–10
caretaking others, 104, 105
Catholicism, 8, 9, 38, 40
chakra, 45, 47, 58, 160
  affected by shadow, 81

E

ego, 141, 149, 159
electromagnetic energy, 28,
    165, 170
electromagnetic vibration.
    See vibration
emotions, 49
    awareness of, 60
    blocked, 66
    chemical aspects, 52
    conflicting, 53, 64, 72,
        80, 115
    effect on health, 56
    most harmful, 53
    negative, 52, 53, 56
    positive, 52, 53, 56
    that lower your vibration,
        50
    that raise your vibration,
        50
energetic blueprint, 79, 164
    definition of, 167
energetic signature, 16, 102,
    129
    definition of, 168
energetic suicide, 128, 129,
    136–40
    definition of, 168
energy center. *See* chakra
energy field, 16, 23, 24, 29,
    32, 45, 48, 49, 53, 54,
    60, 69, 103, 143, 148,
    157, 164, 165

    appearance at time of
        death, 75
    appearance when near
        death, 16, 45
    color of, 49, 127
    definition of, 168
energy system, iii, 27, 28,
    29, 32, 33, 50, 56, 153,
    156, 161
    definition of, 168
energy, as neutral, 63
etheric field. *See* energy field
evil, 125, 128, 159
evolution, spiritual, 147, 150

F

failure, 148, 149
fatigue, 78, *See also* chronic
    fatigue syndrome
fear, 51, 53, 65, 142
    of …. *See* the object of the
        fear, such as death,
        medical intuition, and
        so on
feelings. *See* emotions
fibromyalgia, 16
fight-or-flight response, 53,
    108, 112, 113
flow, 115–17, 116
    definition of, 168
free will, 146

G

generosity, 53

genes, 55, 56, 69
God, 24, 37, 39, 41, 44, 90,
    99, *See also* guidance
    as healer, 163
    connection with, 116,
        123–40, 124, 155
    disconnection from, 80,
        116, 123–40, 124, 126,
        127, 128
    lack of trust in, 125, 126,
        142
    polite indifference to, 50,
        124
God's love, 41, 42
grace, 98, 151
guidance, 3, 36, 39, 40, 44,
    84, 92, 116, 123, 126,
    139, 141–51, 163
    accepting, 96
    definition of, 169
    discernment of, 36
    how it works, 37
    ignoring, 84, 85, 87
    power of, 145
    setting conditions on, 36
    trust in, 146

H

hands-on healing. *See* healing,
    hands-on
happiness, 115
healing, 163, 170
    hands-on, 5, 109, 154,
        163
    our planet, 6

readiness for, 156
spontaneous. *See*
    spontaneous healing
three-step process, 60
heart chakra. *See* chakra,
    heart
heart disease, 45, 53, 73, 119
heaven, 41
helplessness, 51
Higher Power. *See* God
hopelessness, 53, 136

I

illness, iii, 23, 27, 28, 29,
    31, 33, 49, 56, 57, 59,
    63, 64, 66, 116, 135,
    143, 153, 154, 157, 163,
    169
immune system, 28, 52, 53
impotence, 78, 107
incest, 78, 130
infertility, 50
inflammation, 47
inspiration, 128
intimacy, fear of, 50
intuition. *See also* medical
    intuition
    fear of, 23
intuitive readings. *See*
    readings, intuitive

J

Jesus, 6

joy, 41, 44, 116, 118, 128,
  132, 140, 141
  lack of, 154

K

Kubler-Ross, Elisabeth, 127

L

leaving the body, 41
leukemia, 14, 143
Lewis, C. S., 89, 91
Lipton, Bruce, 55, 69
love. *See also* self-esteem
  feeling unworthy of, 59,
    62, 63, 79
  of self, 61, 64
  unconditional, 123, 169,
  unconditional, lack of, 65
LUMOS, 128, 131, 163
lupus, 131

M

magnetics, 76, 77, 86, 118,
  120, 169
  definition of, 169
manipulating others, 51, 66,
  78, 104
medical intuition
  fear of, 17, 22, 23, 36
Medical Intuitives
  assessing, 158
  importance of medical
    training, 159
  qualifications, 158

warning signs, 158
medicine, alternative. *See*
  complementary medicine
migraines, 111–13
mind-body connection, 6,
  49, 52
molestation. *See* abuse or
  incest
money, 71, 107, 109, 116
MS. *See* multiple sclerosis
multiple sclerosis, 1, 4, 16,
  48, 85, 86, 90, 98

N

narrow-mindedness, 53
negative emotions. *See*
  emotions
negative thoughts. *See*
  thoughts
neuropeptides, 52, 63

O

one priority task. *See* priority
  task
ownership, 60, 74

P

parvovirus, 24
personality traits linked to
  disease, 101–13
Pert, Candace, 52
pessimism, 53
Poincaré, Henri, 21

prayer, 3, 36, 37, 39, 50,
  128, 147
predominant belief. *See*
  beliefs, predominant
predominant negative belief.
  See beliefs, predominant
  negative
preventive medicine, 32
priority task, 157
prostate cancer. *See* cancer
prostate problems, 107–10
psychology, 3, 148
psychotherapy, 2, 70, 129,
  162
purpose in life, 117, 119,
  139

R

readings, intuitive
  benefits of, 153
  information received
    during, 157
  of children, 162
  reasons for, 154
  remote, 164
  type of people seeking,
    155
  what happens during, 103,
    157
  who shouldn't seek one,
    156
recipe medicine, 23, 102
relationship, 50, 58, 104,
  116, 121, 155, 157, 169
  desire for, 58, 59

with God, 123, 124, 125,
  135, 146, 150
with self, 111
resistance to disease. *See*
  disease
resonate, 31, 33, 49, 63, 169
  definition of, 169
rheumatoid arthritis, 23, 24

S

SADS. *See* sudden adult death
  syndrome
science, 12, 13, 21, 27, 29,
  55, 57
SDS. *See* sudden death
  syndrome
secrets, as related to breast
  cancer, 104, 144
Self, the. *See* God
self-criticism, 60, 63
self-esteem, 53, 58, 70, 81,
  103, 108, 111, 121, 148,
  See also love, feeling
  unworthy of
  low, 59, 61, 69, 73, 79
  low, reasons for, 64
  raising your, 67
self-fulfilling beliefs. *See*
  beliefs, self-fulfilling
self-sacrifice, 65, 66, 103,
  105
self-worth. *See* self-esteem
serenity, 116, 168
serotonin, 120, 159
sexuality, 107, 109

shadow, 4, 74, 75, 80, 81,
115, 154
definition of, 170
sin, 128
skepticism, 11, 12, 13, 16,
90, 91, 95, 107, 164
soul, 4, 35, 42, 59, 135,
139, 143, 151, 163, 168,
169
soul, 116
Spirit. *See* God
spirit guides, 90
spiritual connection. *See* God,
connection with
spiritual disconnection. *See*
God, disconnection from
spiritual evolution, 147, 150
spiritual responsibility, 124,
125, 165
definition of, 170
spontaneous healing, 5, 6,
98, 145, 154, 163, 164
St. John of the Cross, 83
stress, 46, 52, 69
sudden adult death
syndrome, 16
sudden death syndrome, 38,
See also sudden adult death
syndrome
suffering, as noble, 75, 80,
151
suicide, 130
suicide, energetic. *See*
energetic suicide
surrender, 96

symptoms, 3, 14, 29, 45, 46,
49, 101
synchronicity, 89, 90, 99

T

task. *See* priority task
thoughts, 49
conflicting, 53
effect on health, 56
harmful, 6
negative, 53, 56
positive, 52, 53, 56
positive, that can cause
illness, 57, 65
that lower your vibration,
50
that raise your vibration,
50
three-step healing process, 60
thrombophlebitis, 102
trauma, 70, 74, 112, 154,
163
tribal beliefs, 49, 71, 72, 73,
75, 80, 81, 101–13, 113,
115, 121, 125, 126, 139,
145, 149, 150, 151, 163,
165
definition, 170
effect on health, 72, 101–
13
generic examples of, 71
tribal law, 147, 149
trust, 53
in God or Higher Power,
146

lack of, 112
Type A personalities, 45

U

unconditional love. *See* love, unconditional
unconscious beliefs. *See* beliefs, unconscious

V

varicose veins, 102
vibration, 16, 24, 29, 31, 32, 33
  definition of, 170
  high, 29, 31, 42, 63, 124, 168
  low, 29, 31, 33, 47, 49, 60, 62, 63, 102, 115, 129, 133, 144, 151, 168, 169

low vs. high, 63
lowering your, 30, 53, 54, 56, 72, 73, 137
raising your, 30, 53, 54, 56, 137, 151, 154, 164
victim, 81, 132, *See also* archetype, Victim
  identifying self as, 51, 170
Victim archetype. *See* archetype, Victim

W

Western medicine, 1, 3, 12, 22, 25, 86, 93, 145, 154, 156, 161
workaholics, 74
worrying, 72
worthlessness, feelings of, 62
wounded child, 63

Acknowledgements

I'd like to acknowledge and thank God for unwavering patience with me, for always being available for guidance, and for the gift of Grace.

I also want to acknowledge and thank all those who dared to dream that the world might actually be round, who believed we would walk on the moon, and who risked thinking outside the box to create a better world, especially my brother Tomas for opening his heart and bringing me to Peru; my best friend Rebecca, who has blessed my life in so many ways, for her unconditional love and support and the spunk to not only do shadow work but now teach it with me; and the thousands of clients who have chosen courage over fear.

And last but definitely not least, I thank the talented, brilliant, and inherently gifted Margot Silk Forrest, whom I have affectionately renamed "Mozart" in honor of her creative genius. She has worn many hats during the birthing of this book, including editor, translator, coordinator, and supporter, but most importantly, good friend. I am blessed to have her in my life. It was her dedication, tenacity, and commitment to a grassroots movement whose time has come that brought this book to fruition. Her latest book, *A Short Course in Kindness,* is a testimony to the life she leads. I thank her for her immense help and for making the world a more loving place to live.

What Is the Center
for Spiritual Responsibility?

The Center for Spiritual Responsibility was founded by Christel Nani, RN, Ph.D., as a means of healing what she sees as the worst "disease" on our planet: our perceived separation from God. Nani defines "spiritual responsibility" as taking responsibility for your health and happiness, no matter what illness, wounds, or problems you have – and no matter who or what caused them. Being spiritually responsible is the polar opposite of identifying yourself as a victim.

The Center's primary goal is to enable people to experience a deep spiritual connection that will lead to the healing of physical, emotional, and spiritual illness. Through classes, workshops, individual sessions, vibrational healing, books, and CDs, the Center's clients learn to understand and release their fears of and blocks to God, replacing their unconscious motivations with conscious choices for a shining future.

The Center for Spiritual Responsibility
132 N. El Camino Real, #412
Encinitas, CA 92024
(760) 632-8780
www.ChristelNani.com

About the Author

The Rev. Christel Nani, RN, Ph.D., is a gifted Medical Intuitive who uses her clairvoyant vision to read a person's energetic blueprint with pinpoint accuracy, locating the unconscious traumas, decisions and emotional patterns contributing to a patient's physical, emotional and spiritual illness. Her talent for identifying the one priority task that will reverse these patterns is a true channeling of spiritual goodness.

Nani, an Interfaith minister, is the founder of the Center for Spiritual Responsibility in Encinitas, California, tel. (760) 632-8780. She can also be reached via her website, www.christelnani.com, or her email address, christel@christelnani.com.

Read an Excerpt From
GUIDANCE 24 / 7

Ken had been angry with God when he was diagnosed with can-
cer... I knew that his transition would be gentler and easier if he could re-
connect with God before he went.

Ken and I prayed together for guidance. In my mind's eye, I saw a
picture of him with a big grin on his face driving to various truck stops and
ordering all kinds of pie. I didn't understand the guidance, but I told Ken
what I saw.

His eyes filled with tears as a broad smile spread across his face.

"How could you know," he began, "that my dream is to eat at truck
stops around the country and find the best pie?" Ken was known by his
family and friends as a connoisseur of pie, and he loved to share the great
pie destinations he discovered. In fact, he had often thought of writing the
ultimate pie book.

It was clear that Ken's guidance was to allow himself some joy. This
may seem like a simple task, but for some people it's not. When you get
this kind of guidance, it's God's way of saying, *"You are loved, you are important, you deserve joy, and I want you to be happy."*

That afternoon Ken opened himself to God and wept. He understood now that he was loved and would not die alone. He could fulfill his
dream of going on the great American pie hunt.

When I pray with people, what I hear is their guidance. This is another
word for what I call a person's priority task – the single most important
thing they can do right now to heal, and something that, when accomplished, will untangle a myriad of other problems.

Who would have thought someone's priority task could be so much
fun? But the truth is, I've listened to some great guidance while praying
with others over the years. It included: *"Learn to cook," "Go shopping," "Quit
your job," "Leave your relationship," "Move to Hawaii,"* and, of course, *"Eat pie!"*

Give the Gift of Healing

For additional copies of *Diary of a Medical Intuitive,* or to buy Christel's popular second book, *Guidance 24/7,* go to your favorite local bookstore. You may also call us at (760) 632-8780, or order the books at www.christelnani.com.

For signed copies, please request at the time of ordering.

Christel also has three wonderful CDs, which can be found at www.christelnani.com or www.amazon.com.

- **SPIRITUALITY, PRAYER & GUIDANCE:** Eliminate the misconceptions and conflicts that stand between you and God. Learn how to find your own spiritual path.

- **HEALING THE FIRST THREE CHAKRAS** – The chakras make up the mind-body connection and reveal much about your life. They are highly sensitive barometers of health that become ill before your body does. This CD explains the ways in which your thinking and fears affect your vital first three chakras, and it shows how to heal them.

- **DIARY OF A MEDICAL INTUITIVE** – This riveting presentation includes stories of Christel's clairvoyant gifts not included in the book, the emotional recounting of her healing, and tells an amazing story of what can happen when you follow the guidance that is there for you.